General Information

Cerebrovascular Diseases

Publication data: 'Cerebrovascular Diseases' is published 6 times annually. Volume 5 with 6 issues appears in 1995.

Subscription rates: Subscriptions run for a full calendar year. Prices are given per volume.

Personal subscription:

Subscription	*+ postage and handling*
SFr. 200.–	+ SFr. 10.20 Europe
SFr. 200.–	+ SFr. 15.60 Overseas
US$ 154.00	+ US$ 10.20

(Must be in the name of, billed to, and paid by an individual. Order must be marked 'personal subscription').

Institutional subscription:

Subscription	*+ postage and handling*
SFr. 500.–	+ SFr. 25.50 Europe
SFr. 500.–	+ SFr. 39.– Overseas
US$ 385.00	+ US$ 25.50

Airmail postage: SFr. 36.–, US$ 30.00. (Extra per volume.)

Microforms: Please direct all enquiries and orders to:
University Microfilms Inc.
300 North Zeeb Road, P.O. Box 1346
Ann Arbor, MI 48106-1346 (USA)

Subscription orders: Orders can be placed at agencies, bookstores, directly with the Publisher S. Karger AG, P.O. Box, CH–4009 Basel (Switzerland) or with any of the following distributors:
Deutschland: S. Karger GmbH, Postfach D–79095 Freiburg
France: Librairie Luginbühl 36, bd de Latour-Maubourg, F–75007 Paris
Great Britain, Ireland: S. Karger Publishers 11 Ravenscroft Road Beckenham, Kent BR3 4TP
USA: S. Karger Publishers, Inc. 26 West Avon Road, P.O. Box 529 Farmington, CT 06085
India, Bangladesh, Sri Lanka: S. Karger India Subscription Agency B–5/132 Safdarjung Enclave New Delhi-110029
Japan: Katakura Libri, Inc. 36-9 Hongo 3-chome, Bunkyo-ku, Tokyo 113

Change of address: Both old and new address should be sent to the subscription source.

Advertising: Correspondence and rate requests should be addressed to the Publisher.

Single issues and back volumes: Information can be obtained through the Publisher.

Bibliographic indices: This journal is regularly listed in bibliographic services, including *Current Contents®*.

Book Reviews: Books are accepted for review by special agreement.

KARGER

Official Journal of the European Stroke Council

Cerebrovascular Diseases

KARGER

Printed in Switzerland
on acid-free paper by
Thür AG Offsetdruck, Pratteln

Appears bimonthly:
1 volume per year (6 issues)

Cerebrovascular Diseases

Submission: Only original papers written in English are considered and should be sent to:

J. Bogousslavsky, MD
Service de Neurologie
CHUV
CH–1011 Lausanne (Switzerland)

or:
M.G. Hennerici, MD
Neurologische Klinik
Klinikum Mannheim der
Universität zu Heidelberg
Theodor-Kutzer-Ufer
D–68135 Mannheim (Germany)

Manuscripts should be submitted in quadruplicate (with four sets of illustrations of which one is an original), typewritten double-spaced on one side of the paper, with a wide margin.

Conditions: All manuscripts are subject to editorial review. Manuscripts are received with the explicit understanding that they are not under simultaneous consideration by any other publication. Submission of an article for publication implies the transfer of the copyright from the author to the publisher upon acceptance. Accepted papers become the permanent property of 'Cerebrovascular Diseases' and may not be reproduced by any means, in whole or in part, without the written consent of the publisher. It is the author's responsibility to obtain permission to reproduce illustrations, tables, etc. from other publications.

Arrangement
Title page: The first page of each paper should indicate the title (main title underlined), the authors' names, and the institute where the work was conducted. A short title for use as running head as well as the full address of the author to whom correspondence should be sent are also required.
Full address: The exact postal address complete with postal code must be given at the bottom of the title page. Please also supply Phone, Fax, and E-mail numbers.
Key words: For indexing purposes, a list of 3 – 10 key words in English is essential.
Abstract: Each paper needs an abstract of up to 10 lines.
Small type: Paragraphs which can or must be set in smaller type (case histories, test methods, etc.) should be indicated with a 'p' (petit) in the margin on the left-hand side.
Footnotes: Avoid footnotes. When essential, they are numbered consecutively and typed at the foot of the appropriate page.
Tables and illustrations: Tables and illustrations (both numbered in Arabic numerals) should be prepared on separate sheets. Tables require a heading and figures a legend, also prepared on a separate sheet. For the reproduction of illustrations, only good drawings and original photographs can be accepted; negatives or photocopies cannot be used. When possible, group several illustrations on one block for reproduction (max. size 181 × 223 mm) or provide crop marks. On the back of each illustration, indicate its number, the author's name, and 'top'.

Color illustrations: Up to 6 color illustrations per page can now be integrated with the text at the reduced price of SFr. 600.– / US$ 545.00 per page. Color illustrations are reproduced at the author's expense.

References: In the text identify references by Arabic numerals [in square brackets]. Material submitted for publication but not yet accepted should be noted as 'unpublished data' and not be included in the reference list. The list of references should include only those publications which are cited in the text. Do not alphabetize; number references in the order in which they are first mentioned in the text. The surnames of the authors followed by initials should be given. There should be no punctuation other than a comma to separate the authors. Cite all authors, 'et al' is not sufficient. Abbreviate journal names according to the Index Medicus system. (Also see International Committee of Medical Journal Editors: Uniform requirements for manuscripts submitted to biomedical journals. Br Med J 1988; 296:401–405.)
Examples
(a) Papers published in periodicals: Brenner M, Berberich R, Haass A, Schimrigk K, Pahl J: Platelet scintigraphy in cerebrovascular diseases. Eur Neurol 1989;29:197–201.
(b) Monographs: Hennerici M, Sitzer G, Weger H-D: Carotid Artery Plaques: Pathogenesis – Development – Evaluation – Treatment. Basel, Karger 1988.
(c) Edited books: Abbott NJ, Bundgaard M, Hughes CCW: Morphology of brain microvessels: A comparative approach; in Hammersen F, Messmer K (eds): Cerebral Microcirculation. Prog Appl Microcircul. Basel, Karger, 1990, vol 16, pp 1–20.
Further details: Authors may consult our leaflet 'Rules for the Preparation of Manuscripts', available on request from the Publisher, S. Karger AG, P.O. Box, CH – 4009 Basel (Switzerland).

Galley proofs: Unless indicated otherwise, galley proofs are sent to the first-named author and should be returned with the least possible delay. Alterations made in galley proofs, other than the correction of printer's errors, are charged to the author. No page proofs are supplied.

Reprints: Order forms and a price list for additional reprints are sent with the galley proofs. Orders submitted after the issue is printed are subject to considerably higher prices. Allow five weeks from date of publication for delivery of reprints.

KARGER

Trials for Acute Stroke Therapy

Round Table

Janssen-Cilag
Symposium at the
Fourth European Stroke Conference
Bordeaux, June 1, 1995

Editors
J. Bogousslavsky, Lausanne, Switzerland
P. Koudstaal, Rotterdam, The Netherlands
H.J.M. Barnett, London, Canada

6 tables, 1995

KARGER

Cerebrovascular Diseases
Vol. 5, Supplement 1, 1995

S. Karger
Medical and Scientific Publishers
Basel · Freiburg · Paris · London
New York · New Delhi · Bangkok
Singapore · Tokyo · Sydney

Drug Dosage
The authors and the publisher have exerted every effort to ensure that drug selection and dosage set forth in this text are in accord with current recommendations and practice at the time of publication. However, in view of ongoing research, changes in government regulations, and the constant flow of information relating to drug therapy and drug reactions, the reader is urged to check the package insert for each drug for any change in indications and dosage and for added warnings and precautions. This is particularly important when the recommended agent is a new and/or infrequently employed drug.

P.O. Box, CH–4009 Basel (Switzerland)
Printed in Switzerland on acid-free paper by
Thür AG Offsetdruck, Pratteln
ISBN 3–8055–6228–4

Contents

Cerebrovasc Dis 1995;5(suppl 1):1–2

J. Bogousslavsky

Department of Neurology,
University Hospital, Lausanne,
Switzerland

The Jungle of Acute Stroke Trials, Trialists and Sponsors

Key Words
Acute stroke trials
Drug industry sponsorship
Ethics Committee, Trial design

Abstract
The conducting of effective clinical trials in acute stroke is beset with a range of problems. The entire community involved in such trials (both investigators and sponsors) must attempt to develop high quality protocols; to be responsible for the selection of credible trial centres and to ensure that members of the trial committee are appropriately chosen. The question of who initiates the trial (trialist or sponsor); who collects and analyses the data and the creation of a suitable structure of reimbursement must be addressed. Local Ethics Committees are not suitably equipped for this task which must become the responsibility of a larger, international body.

The field of clinical trials has been developing dramatically over the last few years, to a point which has even justified the creation of specific academic units and journals. Acute stroke has become one of the major target conditions studied in clinical trials. The development is primarily in relation to the tremendous pharmacological advances which have led to many different drugs which are potentially active in acute cerebral ischemia, but it is also due to major progress in our understanding of stroke pathophysiology and aetiology. However, while only few clinicians would disagree that we do need acute stroke trials, the rapid expansion of fundamental and clinical knowledge as well as the multiplication of drugs to be tested has led to confusion and a lack of clarity, in the absence of coordinated efforts by investigators, steering committees and sponsors. Moreover, despite well-designed protocols, this lack of coordinated efforts between the people involved in different trials is particularly frustrating since many investigators and committee members are in fact the same from trial to trial.

In a recent Editorial [1], I asked the question whether this morass might finally lead to 'nirvana', i.e. finding an effective specific therapy for acute stroke in human patients.

If we want to develop an effective consensus, I submit that the following points must be addressed by the community of trialists, investigators and sponsors.

Methodological Aspects

Standard high quality protocols must be developed and adapted from trial to trial. Primary versus secondary endpoints must be agreed upon at an international level. Specific scores and scales to assess improvement should be made more homogenous.

Selection of Centres and Investigators
Clinical trials should be performed in credible centres accepted by appropriate criteria. Participation simulta-

J. Bogousslavsky
Service de Neurologie
CHUV
CH–1011 Lausanne (Switzerland)

1015–9770/95/0057–0001
$8.00/0

neously in several clinical trials with similar protocols and inclusion criteria should be questioned and (within the limit of rules to be established) be avoided. The problem of big compared to small centres, of academic compared to non-academic centres, and of well- established compared to new centres must be discussed.

Selection of Trial Committees' Members

This choice should not be solely the responsibility of the sponsor. The question of the participation of sponsor representatives on trial committees should also be addressed. The simultaneous participation of the same individual on the committees of several similar trials should probably also be addressed by simple rules.

Sponsors

Who selects whom? Is it an interested investigator who should ask for sponsorship or is it a sponsor with a treatment to be tested who should contact investigators? At the moment, the first possibility occurs in most trials financed by non-commercial organizations, while the second takes place in drug company-sponsored trials. Is the discrepancy appropriate or should this practice be modified?

Collection and Analysis of Data

Most trials sponsored by non-commercial organizations have their own central data handling office which independently monitors data handling and to some extent even data analysis. This function is commonly performed, directly or indirectly, by the sponsor in drug company-supported trials. It seems clear that some form of international consensus must be obtained on who should collect, centralize, and analyze the data, and how.

Financial Aspects

This is a delicate and often secret matter. Financial compensation, honoraria, and specific cost reimbursement are not commonly divulged. They may be subject to negotiations between sponsors and investigators, according to centre or investigator prestige or quality, country, and competition between trials. Financial aspects are probably the most obscure and perhaps dangerous part of the stroke trials jungle, and therefore the most difficult aspect of trials to regulate. More overt discussions and hopefully some form of consensus should at least be attempted. I am sure that some people may be shocked by this remark, but I have never fully understood why the randomizing physician is supposed to get an honorarium – often *per capita* – for randomizing patients, while no honorarium is foreseen for the patient who agrees to be randomized. It may be argued that the informed consent given by the patient should be unbiased by financial aspects, but why is it not true for the physician as well? Moreover, in many countries patients may in fact be biased towards acceptance of randomization, since this may be associated with better or cost free follow-up care.

Solutions?

Institutional Ethics Committees are not likely to be helpful in attempts to obviate or solve these problems. Indeed, they are constituted and act at a local level to ensure that the basic respect for colleagues and patient rights will be followed. What we need is a more broad-based and international body to survey and approve multicentre acute stroke trials. This does not need to be a heavily administrative structure. On the contrary, it should be a committee composed of recognized stroke clinicians or scientists without direct interests in the particular trials. This committee should review the protocols and provide a stamp of approval that certain minimal criteria (for the design, monitoring, and sponsorship of the trial, as well as for centres and committee selection, data handling and analysis) have been met. This might limit the overlap between investigators and committees of different trials, allow centralization of information and stimulate networks of qualified centres, but it also could provide an independent body to recommend funding.

In Europe, the European Stroke Council has appointed a subcommittee to make formal proposals on these matters. It is of the utmost importance for the future of acute stroke therapy that we develop better and clearer partnerships between trialists, investigators, sponsors, the pharmaceutical industry, and administrative and licensing offices.

Reference

1 Bogousslavsky J: Acute stroke trials: from morass to nirvana? Celebrovasc Dis 1995;5:3–6.

Cerebrovasc Dis 1995;5(suppl 1):3–11

L.M. Brass

Department of Neurology, Yale University School of Medicine, New Haven, CT, and The Neurology Service of the West Haven Veteran's Affairs Medical Center, West Haven CT, USA

Trial Design Issues: Endpoints and Sample Size

Key Words
Cerebrovascular disorders
Endpoint
Methodology
Randomized clinical trial
Sample size

Abstract
To obtain useful results from clinical trials requires attention to various aspects of the trial design. Important among these is the selection of appropriate endpoints or outcome events. Currently measured endpoints involve determination of impairment, disability or handicap, but these represent three distinct levels of outcome. The importance of psychosocial factors such as social support is being increasingly appreciated as a factor contributing to stroke recovery. In addition, attempts are currently being made to provide suitable measures of the patient's quality of life. There is a considerable lack of clarity and consistency about the meaning and measurement of this variable. Details are given of a new attempt to produce a reliable scoring system to measure quality of life using the patient's own ranking of important items. Intermediate (surrogate) endpoints can be of value but only if they are also clinically relevant. Finally, the question of sample size is important for the design of clinical trials. Many published trials have contained too few patients to exclude the possibility of some undetected therapeutic benefit. Stroke trials of the future would seek to combine a range of endpoints, including biochemistry and clinical observation with assessment of life quality based on the reports of patients themselves.

Since its introduction over 40 years ago, the randomized clinical trial (RCT) has emerged as a powerful and methodologically rigorous scientific paradigm. Its impact is remarkable for the many major therapeutic advances shown to be effective in a RCT, and also for the many therapies shown to be ineffective. Although most physicians feel comfortable with the basic principles of randomized clinical trials, this perception is often wrong. Nearly half of those involved in clinical neurological research have had no formal education in study design and data analysis [1]. In a review of unfunded clinical research grants, 66% had serious deficiencies in methodology [2]. This discussion focuses briefly on endpoints and sample size calculations (table 1). There are many other items critical to a therapeutic trial [3]. The interested reader is referred to several excellent, overview reviews of clinical trial design [3–9].

Endpoints/Outcome Events

Endpoints or outcome events are the variables used to measure the effect of an intervention in a clinical trial. The design, selection, application, and interpretation of

L.M. Brass
Yale Stroke Program, Department of Neurology
P.O. Box 208018
Yale University School of Medicine, 15 York Street
New Haven, CT 06520–8018 (USA)

1015–9770/95/0057–0003
$8.00/0

Table 1. Key items in the design or review of a clinical trial

Element	Issues related to key element
Question	Therapy being tested Dose duration Patient characteristics Criteria for success
Outcome	Primary outcome and definition Secondary outcomes and definitions Complications Censoring
Study Design	Randomization Blinding Control Type of design
Cohort	Target population Screening process Eligibility Cascade Final number of patients randomized
Study Protocol	Follow-up schedule Procedures for call back Number of missed visits
Quality Control	Randomization Evaluation of endpoints Data entry Blindness
Analysis	Statistical methods

endpoints is a complex speciality. A key issue is to be able to draw the appropriate conclusion about the value of a therapy in the shortest amount of time with the fewest number of patients, the least cost, and the least risk to participating individuals.

Data on many clinical variables may be collected during the clinical trial. However, it is important to identify clearly what outcomes will be used to measure efficacy prior to starting the trial. Identifying the primary outcomes guides the trial design, influences the duration of the trial, the frequency of assessment, and details of follow-up examinations. If too many outcomes are examined, some are likely to show a positive effect of a treatment solely by chance (type I error). The outcomes selected should be clinically important and not trivial [10].

The selection of endpoints is not always obvious. Trials of secondary prevention provides a practical example. The goal of a trial of secondary prevention of stroke is not just the prevention of stroke, but the prevention of stroke and death (i.e., stroke free survival) [4]. Death may occur following a stroke and remove individuals who might otherwise, had they lived, have developed a second stroke (known as censoring). Thus, a therapy could reduce the risk of a recurrent stroke, simply by increasing mortality since 'Dead patients cannot have strokes' [11]. Because many deaths following a stroke are related to cardiac disease, and therapies for stroke may influence the heart, the combined endpoint of stroke or death (i.e., stroke free-survival) may be more appropriate for trials than test drugs that purportedly prevent cerebrovascular disease.

The difference in using stroke free survival, as opposed to frequency of recurrent stroke alone, is illustrated in the Ticlopidine-Aspirin Stroke Study which compares ticlopidine and aspirin for the secondary prevention of stroke after a transient ischaemic attack (TIA) or minor stroke [12]. The investigators reported a statistically significant 21% relative risk reduction in recurrent stroke with ticlopidine therapy compared to aspirin. In contrast, when stroke or death (i.e., stroke free survival) was the endpoint, there was only a 12% reduction, and the 95% confidence interval included zero (i.e., the relative risk reduction was not statistically significant).

The endpoints used as judgement criteria for a treatment effect in a clinical trial should also meet several key methodological criteria [13, 14]. They should be: *valid* (able to evaluate the phenomena under study); *reliable* (able to give the same measure when repeated by the same or different investigators); *sensitive* (likely to change with the anticipated benefits of therapy); and *practical* (able to be measured in setting of a clinical trial). The interested reader is referred to several recent review articles [13, 15] and chapters [16–18] for more detailed definitions and discussion.

The World Health Organization's classification of impairment, disability, and handicap covers the basic types of stroke outcome measures that are currently made in clinical trials [13–15, 19].

Impairment refer to a loss of psychological, physiological, or anatomical structure or function. This usually refers to the neurological deficit. It is recorded by items related to the traditional neurological examination. Impairment scales for use with cerebrovascular disease include the NIH stroke scale, the European Stroke Scale [20], the Toronto Stroke Scale [21], Canadian Stroke Scale [22], Orgogozo Scale [23], and Scandinavian Stroke Scale [19] to name just a few.

Disability is the lack or restriction resulting from an impairment. Neurological deficits interact to impair the ability of an individual to perform desired activities. This is a more clinically relevant measure than impairment alone. It is the lack of ability to do something that is especially important after stroke (e.g., not that my leg is weak, but that I cannot walk). Disability is usually measured in stroke trials by the Barthel Index [24] and Functional Independence Measure (FIM) [25].

Handicap is the disadvantage for an individual resulting from their disability. It is usually measured by global outcome scales like the Glasgow Outcome Scale [26] or the Rankin Scale [27].

The characteristics and clinimetric properties of the major stroke scales are reviewed elsewhere [13, 19]. Most of these scales focus on 'hard outcomes' as measured by the neurological examination or derivatives of the neurological examination [14]. They often miss describing the long term functional outcome of an individual patient. Although the handicap scales attempt to categorize functional outcome, measures more focused on the patient, family and their perception of their 'quality-of-life' may help to improve clinical measurements following a stroke. These types of measures form the basis for one of the newer trends within the evaluation of stroke outcome, an increasing emphasis on psychosocial and quality of life measures.

Psychosocial Factors

Many trialists cringe at the prospect of psychosocial outcome measures in therapeutic stroke trials, yet inclusion of this category of endpoints in these measures may help to reduce variability, help better to assess the impact of cerebrovascular disease, improve our understanding of how interventions work, and possibly point the way to new therapies.

There is convincing evidence that a lack of emotional support can reduce survival following myocardial infarction. In a prospective, population-based study, Berkman and colleagues found (after multiple logistic regression analyses), that those with a lack of emotional support were much more likely to die within the first six months following a myocardial infarction [28]. The odds ratio was 2.9 after controlling for severity of myocardial infarction, comorbidity, vascular risk factors, and sociodemographic characteristics.

Higher levels of social support have been associated with faster and more extensive recovery following stroke [29]. Social support may be an important prognostic factor for recurrent stroke or vascular death. Those patients who are socially isolated following a stroke may also be the group most appropriate for therapeutic intervention with enhanced support systems, a strategy currently being tested in a randomized trial (Family Intervention in Recovery from Stroke Trial (FIRST) – NIH NS 32324).

Quality of Life Measurements

Quality of Life is the most comprehensive measure of stroke outcome. It is also the most subjective. The use of the term 'quality of life' is becoming increasingly popular among researchers, quality management personnel, administrations and legislators. Within the past decade, convincing evidence has emerged that quality of life measures can substantially augment other conventional measures of treatment (e.g., blood pressure, stroke, death) in clinical trials [30, 31].

Although many physicians attempt to incorporate these factors intuitively, recommending therapies based on patient preferences, this is usually not taken into account in clinical trials. The practical goal of a clinical trial is to change (improve) patient management. Ultimately, the clinician must decide how to apply the results of a clinical trial based on knowledge of the patient's individual values [32]. This is the practice of the art of medicine, and it is dependent on considering what patients think about a treatment, disease, and themselves.

Although widely quoted, there is a lack of clarity and consistency about the meaning and measurement of quality of life. In a recent critical appraisal of quality of life measurements, only 15% of articles provided a conceptual definition of quality of life [31]. There is little good evidence that current quality of life measurements, even those based on sound psychometric principles, are indicating what clinicians and patients perceive as quality of life.

Few studies even distinguish the overall quality of life measures from health related quality of life (i.e., specifically due to the stroke). Patients with an impaired quality of life should be asked to indicate the relative contribution of their medical illness. For example, a patient with mild neurological deficit following a stroke may report a poor overall quality of life because of a decreased ability to care for a husband with Alzheimer's Disease. If this distinction is ignored, the impact of a disease on the health-related quality of life may be overestimated. Furthermore, the effect of psychosocial intervention by a patient's physicians or health care providers may be grossly underestimated [33].

In addition, most quality of life measures are based on responses to standardized items devised by investigators based on their own perceptions. In only 17% of quality of life studies were patients permitted to give their own global rating for their quality of life [33].

The field is still evolving and holds great potential for augmenting physiological and health status measurements in observational and interventional investigations. Quality of life is based on aspects of life that are especially valued by an individual. People's values differ. The need to move further toward incorporating patients' values and preferences is highlighted by three basic recommendations from Gill and colleagues [33].

Use global ratings. This will help incorporate disparate values and preferences of individual patients.

Rate severity and importance. The severity and importance of elements of quality of life measures should be delineated for specific domains.

Allow supplemental items. Key items may be omitted by investigators on a standard instrument that are likely to be important in the beliefs and values of different groups of people based on factors such as age, race, education, religious beliefs, and psychosocial support. With supplemental items, patients can add factors that may not have been included in the original instrumentation [34, 35].

The issue of relative severity and importance (to the patients) of stroke endpoints is worthy of comment. The clinical impact of vascular endpoints varies greatly, but it is usually not accounted for in clinical trails. For example, although a TIA is often included, appropriately, in some trials of stroke prevention a TIA usually has little long term impact on an individual other than identifying an increased risk for stroke, MI, cognitive decline, or death. Similarly, since stroke is more commonly associated with functional impairment, it may be considered as a less desirable outcome. A treatment which reduced TIA, or alternatively death, at the expense of increasing stroke would not necessarily result in an improvement in patient management. A severe stroke may even be viewed by patients as worse than death [36]. This issue could arise in acute therapeutic trials if statistical significance for a therapy is achieved only by including reduced mortality (i.e., a shift from death to survival with severe disability), even if among those who would have survived there is no net improvement in outcome. A result without regard to severity of endpoints may be used to show that a therapy has an effect, but it is improvements in quality of life that will show that a therapy should be used.

A practical example of the importance of considering severity comes from the recent report of the SPAF II results. For older patients with atrial fibrillation, the number of strokes was slightly reduced with warfarin therapy (compared with aspirin). However, the rate of disabling strokes was *higher* among those taking warfarin. Although reviewing severity of endpoints is not as helpful in understanding *how* warfarin changes the rate of stroke (looking at stroke type may be), it is very helpful to deciding *whether* warfarin therapy should be used [37].

Dr. Thomas Gill and I are collaborating, along with other colleagues in New Haven, in a pilot study of quality of life assessment following stroke [31]. It is worth noting that different strategies are used with clinimetric and psychometric methods of constructing indexes and rating scales [38]. For example, a single psychometric measure such as depression, may be based on many items, whereas clinimetric strategies measure many attributes within a single index (such as quality of life). Because of factors mentioned earlier, patients are asked to give two global ratings, one for their overall quality of life, the other for health (stroke) related quality of life. An example of part of our questionnaire is shown as a visual analogue scale (table 2).

In addition, based on the recommendation listed above, patients are also asked during open ended interviews to identify problems, both general and specific, related to their stroke. This approach is motivated, in part, by one of the most basic questions in clinical care, 'How are you?' Attention is paid to items they perceive as important for their quality of life and not a reiteration of their neurological deficit. (For example, not accepting 'my arm is weak', but rather assessing the impact 'I can no longer take care of myself and I feel guilty that my son has to miss work to help me prepare my meals').

This can help define new areas of concern to patients. For example in similar work with judging the success of total hip replacement, traditional scoring systems had focused on an important, but limited range of items [34]. The ability to maintain pain-free sexual activity was identified as an important outcome to a significant portion of patients undergoing hip replacement. This type of information can not only improve the performance of clinical scoring systems, it can also improve patient selection, counselling, and expand the focus of rehabilitation programmes.

Finally, to help ensure complete ascertainment, patients in our project review a standardized list of problems commonly encountered following stroke. They may then select items not mentioned during their open ended interview.

The key to this process is to be able to use the information. Following the interview, all items are ranked by patients in order of importance for the construction of a scoring system. Quality of life scores can then be created based on the five more important, patient-specific, quality-of-life items [31].

Other scoring systems, similarly constructed and based on items selected by individual patients have been used successfully in assessing patients with chronic lung disease [39], rheumatoid arthritis [40], low back pain, and hip replacement [34, 35]. These patient specific scores are often more responsive to change than conventional indexes [35, 40, 41]. This latter characteristic may be especially useful for assessing patients following stroke where the scoring in ordinal handicap systems is fairly crude (and hence less sensitive to change).

Table 2. Sample global outcome questions for measuring quality of life following stroke

We are interested in knowing about your overall quality of life in general at the present time. Place an 'X' on the line below indicating where on a scale of 1 to 100 your would rate your overall quality of life, where 0 is 'As bad as it can get' and 100 is 'As good as it can get'

0 As bad as it can get	100 As good as it can get

Now we would like to know how much your stroke has specifically affected your quality of life as it is right now. Place an 'X' on the line below indicating where on a scale of 0 to 100 you would rate the impact of your stroke on your quality of life, where 0 is 'No impact', and 100 is 'Very large impact'

0 No impact	100 Very large impact

New Approaches to Humanistic Phenomena

As mentioned above, quality of life measures are a uniquely personal perception, representing how a person feels about their health status and nonmedical aspects of their lives. New methods are evolving for studying other humanistic clinical phenomena in clinical care. They include methods for studying for patients' goals (as described above), and also physicians' decision making behaviours, and clinical outcomes in the care of patients. The newer methods are particularly concerned with the role of crucial personal and clinical phenomena that generally have been omitted from most studies in health care research such as patients' symptoms, function, and aspirations for a level of quality-of-life, and also doctor's preferences in health care and doctor-patient interactions. These humanistic factors can have paramount effects on patient satisfaction, prognostic estimations, therapeutic choices, and long-term outcomes. Nevertheless, because suitable systems of taxonomy have not been developed to collect and classify the pertinent information, it has seldom been obtained and analyzed. This topic is, in part, an outgrowth of the quality of life work mentioned above and pilot work is beginning with the Veteran Affairs Medical Center at West Haven, CT (VA Merit Review SDR #93–001: Concato J, Brass LM, and Feinstein AR, Principal Investigators).

Intermediate (Surrogate) Endpoints

In animal studies of neuroprotective agents, few animals are needed to demonstrate an effect because the animals are usually sacrificed and a measure of the volume of infarction can be done which is easily quantitated and highly reproducible. Because of the great variation in clinical measures following stroke, with the associated large number of patients and expense required to test new therapies, there has been an increasing interest in the use of intermediate or surrogate endpoints.

Ideally, intermediate endpoints should be safe, inexpensive, reliable, and correlate with meaningful outcomes in the disease processes likely to be effected by treatment. The use of surrogate endpoints is common in some areas of medicine. The treatment of cholesterol and high blood pressure, and their use as endpoints in therapeutic trials, is appropriate given the close association of these factors with myocardial infarction and vascular death.

For stroke, location and size of infarction are two of the main determinants of neurological impairment. A number of methods have been proposed to quantitate the lesion with CT imaging [42]. However, there is significant variation with different operators and between centres.

Newer brain imaging techniques, including advanced magnetic resonance (MR) techniques, are opening up new views of the brain [43]. MR techniques have already been applied in clinical trials for other brain diseases. For example, signal abnormalities present on brain MRI at the time of development of optic neuritis are associated

Table 3. Sample size for dichotomous variables (above) and continuous variables (below)

$$n = \left[\frac{Z_{\alpha/2}\sqrt{2P(1-P)} + Z_{\beta}\sqrt{P_e(1-P_e) + P_c(1-P_c)}}{P_e - P_c} \right]^2$$

$$n = \frac{2\sigma^2 (Z_{\alpha/2} + Z_{\beta})^2}{\delta^2}$$

Where n = sample size (for each group); $Z_{\alpha/2}$ = critical Z value for alpha; Z_{β} = critical Z value for beta; P_c = portion of responders in the control group; P_e = portion of responders in the experimental treatment group; P = the proportion of responders in both groups; σ = weighted standard deviation in the control group; and δ = difference in means between the control and experimental groups.

with risk of developing multiple sclerosis. Therapy with an intravenous methylprednisolone regimen reduces the rate of new demyelinating events [44]. If the development, and lack of development, of these lesions is reliably associated with the development or progression of multiple sclerosis, then a change in the appearance of sequential MRI studies may be appropriate to demonstrate a beneficial effect of a proposed therapy [45].

MRI diffusion mapping also holds potential as an intermediate outcome for clinical trials of acute stroke therapy [46]. Reductions in the apparent diffusion coefficient of water following ischemic injury may provide information about the potential for reversal with reperfusion [47]. Similarly, with improvements in MR techniques and computational analysis, measures of the volume of infarction can be made with increasing precision. There may also be other effective measures such as N-acetyl aspartate or brain lactate [48, 49].

Intermediate outcome measures are certainly appealing for clinical trials. However, important questions remain. For example, if there is a 5% reduction in stroke volume, but no change in neurological outcome, how much effort, expense, or risk should be undertaken when introducing a therapy into clinical management? [50] There are also important methodological issues that must be addressed. Even if an intermediate endpoint is used with one acute therapy, it may not be appropriate for use with others. For example, DWI measured at 4 hours following reperfusion therapy may accurately predict long-term outcome and can be used as an intermediate outcome. For other agents like anti-ICAM (which may inhibit white cell migration into an infarction), the main effect being blocked (i.e., inflammatory) may not reach its peak for several days. It seems unlikely that early DWI measures would be able to predict effectiveness of this class of therapy.

It is also worth considering that many of the currently used stroke scales in acute therapeutic trials are really intermediate outcome measures for an individual's ultimate quality of life. The decision to use a new therapy should remain based on whether it helps make patients better. This is true whether the effect is measured by a clinical stroke outcome measure or an MR intermediate outcome. A quote attributed to Gertrude Stein summarizes much of the design and interpretation of clinical trials [5]. 'For a difference to be a difference, it has to make a difference.'

Sample Size

Endpoints strongly impact on the number of patients needed to test a new therapy. The following basic sample size equations [51] include several assumptions beyond the scope of this discussion, but illustrate some of the effects of endpoint selection on sample size (table 3).

The Z values for alpha and beta are quantitative values determined by the selection of levels for type I and type II errors. These 'errors' reflect the random fluctuation seen whenever the same experiment (including clinical trial) is repeated several times. A trial with a beneficial therapy, may by chance show no 'beneficial' effect. In setting up a clinical trial of a new therapy, the investigators should decide how willing they are to miss potentially significant results. This is the type I (also called alpha) error where the results of the trial suggest that there is a difference when the true answer is no difference (i.e., false positive). This could lead to accepting the new agent as more effective, when it is not. Conventionally, a value of 5% is usually set (and Z_{α} = 1.96 (two-sided)). A type II (beta) error occurs when the results of a trial show no effect of a therapy when this is wrong (false negative). This means that an effective therapy is rejected as being ineffective. Conventionally, the probability of making a type II error is usually set at less than 0.20 (and Z_{β} = 0.84 (one sided)). 'Power' is the probability that it will detect a clinically important difference if one exists. The power is defined as $(1-\beta)$.

Interestingly, nearly all trials report a p value (reflecting the changes for a type 1 error), yet the beta value is not reported in most clinical studies. The importance of this lies in our assuming that a 'negative' trial means that a therapy is ineffective. Freiman and colleagues reviewed negative randomized controlled trials looking to see how many had a greater than 90% chance of having missed a therapeutic benefit of 25%. In 80% (57/71) of studies, there was an inadequate sample to exclude what most would consider to be an important treatment effect [52].

Two key points from sample size equations are relevant here:

Difference in treatment. In the equations, it is the absolute difference (not the relative difference) that impacts on the sample size. This means that a relative risk reduction of a third (say in recurrent stroke or death) from 15% (controls) to 10% (in the treated group) will require over three times as many patients as a third reduction from a rate of 45% (controls) to 30% (treated) [53].

Variation in the measurement of outcomes. This strongly impacts on sample size with the number of patients required being proportional to the square of the standard deviation. This means that selecting endpoints with even modest reductions in variability can dramatically reduce the required sample size.

Conclusions

Endpoints are a critical aspect of planning, performing, interpreting and applying clinical trials. Which stroke scales or indices are the most useful will become easier to determine once effective neuroprotective or reperfusion therapies exist and direct comparisons can be made in that setting. Given the high correlation between most existing measures, it seems unlikely that one will be dramatically better than another.

The great promise in endpoints, however, comes from newer stroke outcome measures based on better quantitating the effect of stroke on quality-of-life and biochemical measures in vivo. That these categories of endpoints will require the integration of molecular phenomena and time-honoured bedside techniques should be eminently rewarding to those who recognize the need for a holistic approach to stroke clinimetrics [54].

References

1 Clinical Research Subcommittee of the Scientific Issues Committee of the American Academy of Neurology. Status of clinical research in neurology: Neurology 1995;45:839–845.
2 Cuca JM: NIH grant applications for clinical research: reasons for poor ratings or disapproval. Clin Res 1983;31:453–461.
3 Ellenberg JH: Clinical trials. Neurologic Clinics 1990;8:15–30.
4 Brass LM: The Design and Appraisal of Randomized Clinical Trials in Cerebrovascular Disease and CNS Trauma. Research Publications – Association for Research in Nervous & Mental Disease 1993;71:239–263.
5 Feinstein AR: Clinical Epidemiology: the Architecture of Clinical Research. Philadelphia: Saunders, 1985.
6 Capildeo R, Orgogozo JM: Methodology of Clinical Trials in Neurology: Vascular and Degenerative Brain Disease. London: MacMillan Press Ltd., 1988.
7 Friedman LM, Furberg CD, DeMets DL: Fundamentals of Clinical Trials. Littleton, Massachusetts: PSG Publishing Co, Inc., 1985.
8 Spilker B: Guide to Clinical Trials. New York: Raven Press, Ltd., 1991.
9 Pocock SJ: Clinical Trials: A Practical Approach. New York: John Wiley & Sons, 1983.
10 Laupacis A, Sackett DL, Roberts RS: An assessment of clinically useful measurements of the consequences of treatment. N Engl J Med 1988;318:1728–1733.
11 Sackett DL, Gent M: Controversy in counting and attributing events in clinical trials. N Engl J Med 1979;301:1410–1412.
12 Hass WK, Easton JD, et al: A randomized trial comparing ticlopidine hydrochloride with aspirin for the prevention of stroke in high-risk patients. N Engl J Med 1989;321:501–507.
13 Orgogozo JM, Dartigues JF: Methodology of clinical trials in acute cerebral ischemia. Cerebrovasc Dis 1991;1 (suppl 1):100–111.
14 Lyden PD, Lau GT: A critical appraisal of stroke evaluation and rating scales. Stroke 1991;22:1334–1352.
15 van Gijn J: Measurement of outcome in stroke prevention trials. Cerebrovasc Dis 1992;2 (suppl 1):23–34.
16 Maurer W, Commenges D: Choice of analysis of judgement criteria. In: Capildeo R, Orgogozo JM ed. Methods in Clinical Trials in Neurology. London: MacMillan, 1988:29–55.
17 Feinstein AR: Clinimetrics. New Haven: Yale University Press, 1987.
18 Feinstein AR, Josephy BR, Wells CK: Scientific and clinical problems in indexes of functional disability. Ann Int Med 1986;105:413–420.
19 Hantson L, DeKeyser J: Neurological scales in the assessment of cerebral infarction. Cerebrovasc Dis 1994;4 (suppl 2):7–14.
20 Hantson L, De Weerdt W, De Keyser J, et al: The European Stroke Scale. Stroke 1994;25: 2215–2219.
21 Norris JW: Steroid therapy in acute cerebral infarction. Arch Neurol 1976;33:69–71.
22 Côté R, Hachinski VC, Shurvell BI, Norris JW, Wolfson C: The Canadian Neurological Scale: A preliminary study in acute stroke. Stroke 1986;17:731–737.
23 Orgogozo JM: Evaluation of treatments in ischemic stroke patients. In: Amery WK, Bousser MG, Rose FC ed. Clinical Trial Methodology in Stroke. London: Balliere Tindall, 1989.
24 Mahoney FJ, Barthel DW: Functional evaluation: The Barthel index. Md State Med J 1965; 14:61–65.
25 Grimby G: Quantification of disability after stroke. Cerebrovasc Dis 1994;4 (suppl 2):15–18.
26 Jennet B, Bond M: Assessment of outcome after severe brain damage: A practical scale. Lancet 1975;i:480–484.
27 Rankin J: Cerebral vascular accidents in patients over the age of 60: Prognosis. Scot Med J 1957;2:200–215.
28 Berkman LF, Leo-Summer L, Horwitz RI: Emotional support and survival after myocardial infarction. Ann Int Med 1992;117:1003–1009.
29 Glass TA, Matchar DB, Belyea M, Feussner JR: Impact of social support on outcome in first stroke. Stroke 1993;24:64–70.
30 Croog SH, Levine S, Testa MA, et al: The effects of antihypertensive therapy on the quality of life. N Engl J Med 1986;314:1657–1664.
31 Gill TM: Quality of life assessment. J Roy Soc Med 1995 [in press].
32 Guyatt GH, Cook DJ: Editorial comments: appraisal of the quality of quality-of-life measures, JAMA 1994;272:630–631.
33 Gill TM, Feinstein AR: A critical appraisal of the quality of quality-of-life measurements. JAMA 1994;272:619–626.

34 Wright JG, Rudicel S, Feinstein AR: Ask patients what they want. Evaluation of individual complaints before total hip replacement. J Bone Joint Surg [Br] 1994;76-B:229–234.
35 O'Boyle CA, McGee H, Hickey A, O'Malley K, Joyce CR: Individual quality of life in patients undergoing hip replacement. Lancet 1992;339: 1088–1091.
36 Solomon NA, Glick MA, Russo CJ, Lee J, Schulman KA: Patient preferences for stroke outcomes. Stroke 1994;25:1721–1725.
37 Stroke Prevention in Atrial Fibrillation Investigators: Warfarin versus aspirin for prevention of thromboembolism in atrial fibrillation: Stroke Prevention in Atrial Fibrillation II Study. Lancet 1994;343:687–691.
38 Wright JG, Feinstein AR: A comparative contrast of clinimetric and psychometric methods for constructing indexes and rating scales. J Clin Epidemiol 1992;45:1201–1218.
39 Guyatt GH, Berman LB, Townsend M, Pugsley SO, Chambers LW: A measure of quality of life for clinical trials in chronic lung disease. Thorax 1987;42:773–778.
40 Tugwell P, Bombardier C, Buchanan WW, et al: Methotrexate in rheumatoid arthritis. Impact of quality of live assessed by traditional standard-item and individualized patient preference health status questionnaires. Arch Int Med 1990;150:59–62.
41 Guyatt GH, Townsend M, Pugsley SO, et al: Bronchodilators in chronic air-flow limitation. Effects of airway function, exercise capacity, and quality of life. Am Rev Resp Dis 1987;135: 1069–1074.
42 Brott T, Marler JR, Olinger CP, Adams HP, Tomsick T, Barsan WG, Biller J, Eberle R, Hertzberg V, Walker M: Measurement of acute cerebral infarction: lesion size by computed tomography. Stroke 1989;20:871–875.
43 Prichard JW, Brass LM: New anatomical and functional imaging methods. Ann Neurol 1992; 32:395–400.
44 Fisher CM: Some neuro-ophthalmological observations. J Neurol Neurosurg Psychiatry 1967;30:383–401.
45 McDonald WI, Thompson AJ: Are magnetic resonance findings predictive of clinical outcome in therapeutic trials in multiple sclerosis? The dilemma of interferon-b. Ann Neurol 1994;36:14–18.
46 Minematsu K, Fisher M, Li L, Davis MA, Knapp AG, Cotter RE, McBurney RN, Sotak CH: Effects of a novel NMDA antagonist on experimental stroke rapidly and quantitatively assessed by diffusion-weighted MRI. Neurology 1993;43:397–403.
47 Hasegawa Y, Fisher M, Latour LL, Dardzinski BJ, Sotak CH: MRI diffusion mapping of reversible and irreversible ischemic injury in focal brain ischemia. Neurology 1994;44:1484–1490.
48 Graham GD, Balmire AM, Rothman DL, Brass LM, Fayad PB, Petroff OAC, Prichard JW: Early temporal variation of cerebral metabolites after human stroke: A proton magnetic resonance spectroscopy study. Stroke 1993; 24:1891–1896.
49 Graham GD, Kalach P, Blamire AM, Brass LM, Fayad PB, Prichard JM: Clinical correlates of proton magnetic resonance spectroscopy findings after acute cerebral infarction. Stroke 1995;26:225–229.
50 Raju TNK, Langenberg P, Sen A, Aldana O: How much better is good enough? The magnitude of treatment effect in clinical trials. AJDC 1992;146:407–411.
51 Young MJ, Bresnitz EA, Strom BL: Sample size nomograms for interpreting negative clinical studies. Ann Int Med 1983;99:248–251.
52 Freiman JA, Chalmers TC, Smith H, Kuebler RR: The importance of beta, the Type II error and sample size in the design and interpretation of the randomized control trial. N Engl J Med 1978;299:690–694.
53 Spence JD, Donner A: Problems in design of stroke treatment trials. Stroke 1982;13:94–99.
54 Feinstein AR: Basic clinimetric science in the 21st century. In: Hardy MA, Kinne RKH ed. Biology and Medicine into the 21st Century. New York:Karger, 1991:178–195.

Discussion

H.J.M. Barnett (Ontario, Canada): On the question of reducing the sample size, the absolute and relative risk prediction means that an inadequate sample size to give an absolute risk reduction will create problems.

L.M. Brass (West Haven, USA): Yes. We routinely report the p value, the chances of there being a difference. What is rarely recorded in clinical trials is the beta value, the chance that we have erroneously missed a therapeutic difference. In the *New England Journal of Medicine* a few years ago this problem was reviewed. It was found that of negative reports within well respected journals, nearly 80% of reports that were negative had a greater than 90% probability of missing a 25% improvement in the therapy which was hence recorded as negative. Most trials that do not record a positive result are not convincing evidence that there is no effect of that medication.

H.J.M. Barnett: The absence of proof is not the proof of absence.

L.M. Brass: Absolutely.

K. Prasad (New Delhi, India). I fully agree with you that quality of life measures are probably important endpoints. But most people who have worked with quality of life measures, with a few exceptions, did not attempt to measure what actually is clinically important. I also disagree with your view on intermediate outcomes. We are looking for clinically relevant outcomes and most of the time, intermediate outcomes are not clinically relevant.

L.M. Brass: I think that intermediate outcomes are only useful if they help predict clinically important ones. I'm not particularly interested in lowering someone's lactate as an intermediate measure unless I know that makes their life better. Quality of life measures can be made quantitative. At the end of the quality of life assessment that we are developing, we have three types of information. Global and health related information is measured on some type of 0–100 scale, and relates to their neurologic deficit. We include open-ended questions, where patients tell us what is wrong, and then a list of standardized items that other patients have reported and those based on our experience after strokes. After they have completed those three issues, we then ask them to identify the five most important ones from the list, and attach a relative value to each. Those five items are combined into a single composite score, which can actually perform very well as a clinical variable. In trials of COPD where we all think that the forced expliratory volume, vital capacity, and blood oxygenation capacity represents hard data, this type of composite quality of life measure was more sensitive to detecting change than those other standard hard measures. It can be done in a methodologically rigorous way.

P. Sandercock (Edinburgh, Scotland): I am not sure that there are any intermediate endpoints that we would all agree are appropriate for use in stroke patients yet. Secondly, as we learn from the cardiology field, the dangers of intermediate endpoints are substantial. For example, there were agents which suppress cardiac arrhythmias in acute myocardial infarction that looked highly promising, but actually increased mortality. The intermediate endpoint, the frequency of arrhythmias, was seriously misleading. The same is true for the safety of treatments. There was evidence from the vascular patency studies with thrombolysis in acute myocardial infarction that tPA produced better earlier patency, but the clinically important outcome was cerebral bleeding, and that does appear to be rather more frequent with tPA. The intermediate endpoint was again seriously misleading. I do think we have to be careful, in acute stroke, about which intermediate endpoints we examine.

L.M. Brass: I absolutely agree. I think that an intermediate endpoint which may be appropriate for one trial may not be appropriate for another. For example diffusion-weighted imaging which may be appropriate at 6 hours for an NMBA blocker, may not be appropriate for an anti-ICAM agent, which may not begin to have its effect for several days.

N. Bornstein (Tel Aviv, Israel): I fully agree that we need to measure the quality of life. But for each one of us the quality of life is different. For a musician, a very mild impairment with a clumsy hand may reduce the quality of life is zero, where for a carpenter it probably won't make any difference. You need homogeneous groups to produce a standardized measure of quality of life for each individual.

L.M. Brass: By allowing patients themselves to decide what is important, you can compare an accountant who can no longer add figures in his head with a musician who no longer has dexterity. Each of them will rate their most important five items differently. By allowing patients to attach relative values you can minimise the problem. This has worked with other types of measures. After hip fracture, while increased walking was important to some patients, sexual activity was more important to others.

Cerebrovasc Dis 1995;5(suppl 1):12–15

H.C. Diener[a]
L. Hantson[b]

[a] Department of Neurology, University of Essen, Germany
[b] Clinical Research and Development, Janssen Research Foundation, Titusville, NJ, USA

Clinical Trials for Acute Stroke Therapy: Phase II versus Phase III Trials

Key Words
Clinical trial methodology
Acute stroke studies
Phase II clinical trials
Phase III clinical trials
Drug safety
Drug efficacy

Abstract
Trial methodology for clinical trials in stroke depends upon the specific purposes of the particular trial. Phase II clinical investigation is intended to include early controlled clinical trials designed to demonstrate safety, to gather information on the pharmacokinetic profile of the investigational drug and to establish first proof of efficacy. Phase III clinical trials are expanded controlled trails. They are performed after efficacy has been established, at least to a certain degree, and are intended to gather additional evidence on efficacy, plus further evidence of safety and tolerance.

Trial methodology in acute stroke studies has been the subject of many discussions. Getting agreement on trial design, eligibility criteria, primary efficacy parameters, neurological scales and study sample size is not always easy to accomplish. The choice of these methodological aspects obviously depends upon the specific features or purposes of a particular trial. A pragmatic study with an intention-to-treat design and analysis will significantly differ from an explanatory approach. Whether a pragmatic or explanatory design is preferred often depends on the stage of clinical development of the experimental compound.

A clinical trial can be defined as a prospective study in human subjects, either in patients or non-patient volunteers [1]. The purpose of a clinical trial is to provide valid evidence of the effects of medical therapy and in so doing will study areas such as absorption, distribution, metabolism and excretion of drug. Later, the controlled clinical trial, more precisely defined as a prospective study comparing the effect and value of intervention(s) against a control (standard treatment or placebo) in human subjects, is important in accurate determination of therapeutic effects. Clinical trials may be classified as therapeutic, interventional or preventative trials, depending on whether the objective is to treat, reduce the incidence of, or prevent disease. Therapeutic trials are classified into Phase I, II, III and IV, though in practice companies are tending to move away from doing studies in a strictly chronological fashion and tend to have integrated plans which incorporate key decision points during development. The nature and methodological aspects of Phase II and Phase III trials in the acute treatment of an ischaemic stroke are summarised below.

Phase II and III Trial Objectives

Phase II clinical investigation is intended to include early controlled clinical trials designed to demonstrate efficacy and safety and to gather information on the pharmacokinetic profile of the investigational drug. Phase II studies can be divided into early and late Phase II trials.

H.C. Diener
Department of Neurology
University of Essen
Hufelandstrasse 55
D–45122 Essen (Germany)

1015–9770/95/0057–0012
$8.00/0

Early Phase II trials are mainly focused on the safety and pharmacokinetic profile of the experimental compound in the target population (i.e., ischaemic stroke patients). The main objective of a late Phase II study is to further investigate the safety and pharmacokinetic aspects of the drug and to establish first proof of efficacy. At this time point of development a decision should be made whether or not the experimental drug should be further developed. An efficacious drug may be toxic or might have a high cost/benefit ratio. Phase III clinical trials are the expanded control trials. There are performed after efficacy has been basically established, at least to a certain degree, and are intended to gather additional evidence of efficacy, plus further evidence of safety and tolerance.

It is remarkable that the majority of the compounds that are currently in Phase III development for the acute treatment of stroke lack positive Phase II data e.g. efficacy. Indeed, obtaining positive efficacy data in a Phase II study with a small sample size is difficult to achieve. However, a trend for superiority should at least be found before large scale Phase III trials are initiated.

Phase II trials are important for dose selection in humans and are therefore most frequently dose-finding studies. These studies aim at the determination of appropriate dose ranges and regimens and clarification of dose/response relations, in order to prove an optimal background for the design of wider therapeutic trials. It is desirable to ascertain the range of effectiveness. Thus, the lowest effective dose and, when feasible, the highest safe and effective dose are determined. Phase III trials should be conducted with a limited number of doses, preferably only one. Safe dosage regimens, that preferably result in plasma/brain levels that were neuroprotective in animal stroke models, should be selected. However, only a limited number of compounds in development attain plasma or brain levels that are neuroprotective in animal models.

Study Design

Normally, early Phase II studies are performed in an open-label fashion with a limited number of closely monitored patients. In view of the natural history of recovery after a stroke, the difficulty of making a good outcome prognosis and the lack of an effective treatment for acute stroke, efficacy studies (i.e., late Phase II and Phase III studies) are performed placebo- controlled. The situation is more complicated in stroke prevention. There is no doubt that antiplatelet agents are effective in the prevention of stroke after transient ischaemic attacks (TIA) and stroke [2]. As long as the ideal dose of acetylsalicylic acid (ASA) is not defined and the risk/benefit for different doses is not finally clarified, it is difficult to decide which ASA dose should serve as control against a new substance.

Although randomization of patients among various treatment groups is generally satisfactory when one is treating the same disease, it is often preferable to stratify patients prior to grouping (e.g. inclusion time $>$ or <6 hours). This will help to ensure balance of treatment groups for major prognostic factors and appropriate analysis of results among subgroups that may be more or less responsive to the drug. In view of the small sample size of a late Phase II study, matching might be more important than in a larger scaled Phase III trial. In Phase III trials, matching of patients might be accomplished without any further specific effort. However, since an experimental substance for stroke treatment will only be effective in a certain time window (several hours), stratification according to inclusion time is highly recommended in both Phase II and Phase III studies. In every day practice, however, most stroke patients arrive in the hospital when the time window has expired and would therefore not be eligible for treatment. The result of the trial might finally be positive, but cannot be generalized for the whole population of stroke patients.

Study Population

Phase II studies will seldom go beyond 100–200 patients on drug, all under rigidly controlled protocols. In view of the high variability in recovery, these numbers are too small to detect a statistically significant difference. The trends, if any, however, allow one to decide whether further trials are justified. The sample size of a Phase III study is much larger. The majority of these protocols include 500–1500 patients. One Phase III (or Phase IV?) study targeting 20,000 patients is currently being conducted [3]. In Phase III studies, the number of patients should permit the demonstration of a statistically significant difference between the control and active group. This can be accomplished by means of a power calculation. This calculation should be based upon the compound's effect as seen in earlier Phase II studies. Namely, the greater the effect of the compound, the smaller the probability of type II error for a given sample size and alpha. Thus, for a specified sample size and alpha, the statistical test will detect large differences more easily than small ones. As the sample size gets larger, the probability of type II error gets smaller for a given difference in means and alpha. Thus to detect the specified difference between control and active treatment, we make the test more powerful by increasing the sample size.

A homogeneous patient population should be selected for Phase II studies, allowing one to investigate the efficacy, safety and pharmacokinetics in a limited number of patients. Patients selected for early Phase II studies should be (as much as possible) free of haematologic, hepatic, renal, cardiac or other serious disease, to avoid possible interference with assessment of safety of the investigational drug. If feasible, the concomitant medication should be limited. In view of the aetiology of stroke (e.g., the important role of any underlying cardiac disease), this is very difficult to accomplish. In late Phase II studies, in order to establish first proof of efficacy in a small group of patients, a homogeneous patient population with respect to outcome should also be aimed for. This can be achieved by including eligibility criteria based on prognostic factors for outcome. Generally the circumstance of a Phase III trial should be as close as possible to normal conditions of use. A more heterogenous patient population (and other concomitant diseases or underlying cardiac pathologies) may be targeted since they would be expected to be more representative of certain segments of the population who will be receiving the investigational drug following approval for marketing.

Assessments

In Phase II, the safety assessments and laboratory tests will be performed more frequently than in Phase III studies. The frequency will vary with the nature and safety of the drug. For some drugs (i.e., NMDA-antagonists [4]) daily supervision may be necessary during trial medication, despite the stage of clinical development.

Efficacy of the experimental compound can be measured at different hierarchical levels: impairment, disability and handicap. Impairment is the direct neurophysiological consequence of the underlying pathology. Disability refers to the functional consequences of any impairment, whereas handicap is the social and societal consequence of the disease. In contrast to a functional and handicap scale, a neurological scale is used in both Phase II and Phase III trials for describing the patient's base-line characteristics in terms of stroke severity, for matching of the treatment groups for prognostic factors and for defining specific protocol criteria. This scale should be reliable, valid, sensitive and easy to use. The items that comprise the scale should be prognostic for outcome and be specific for the type of stroke investigated [5]. A neurological scale evaluates a drug's effect more directly than a functional or handicap scale, without the complications of motivation, support, family, social context, etc. It might therefore be more specific and sensitive to a treatment effect than a disability or a handicap scale. Claim of a compound's effect in small sampled Phase II efficacy trials could therefore rely more on a neurological scale. A functional scale should be assessed in Phase II as well. The large sampled Phase III trials will primarily focus on the patient's functional ability at outcome and the sample size will be calculated on the effect seen in earlier Phase II studies.

In addition to all these different types of scales, mortality can be used as an efficacy parameter. Reducing mortality is indeed a clinical important outcome. However, a reduction in mortality should not result in an increased morbidity. The major advantage of mortality is that it is a valid, sensitive and reliable endpoint.

Phase II studies should be performed by a limited number of investigators who are considered experts in the particular disease categories to be treated and/or in evaluation of drug effects on the disease process. Phase III trials should try to mimic real life situation and should (in view of the required sample size) be performed as multi-centre and often multi-national investigations.

Outcomes Research

The objectives of Outcomes Research during Phases II and III differ substantially. Phase II can be considered as the planning and development phase, whereas Phase III is the implementation phase.

One of the most frequent mistakes in Outcomes Research is that people start planning too late. In fact, one should start no later than late Phase II. The extent of the Outcomes Research data needed in support of the product's pricing and reimbursement as well as formulary acceptance will be examined. This involves a thorough analysis of the environmental factors. In parallel, the research hypotheses regarding the product's impact on Economic and Quality of Life (QoL) parameters have to be defined. Secondly, information on the natural history of stroke, on medical practices, treatment patterns and associated resource use will be gathered through epidemiological and cost-of-illness studies. This information will help to assess the scope and the nature of the Economic and QoL endpoints of importance for ischaemic stroke. The above information allows for a development of the product's Outcomes Research strategy. Thirdly, an Economic (resource use) questionnaire will be developed and a QoL battery will be selected. The appropriate economic/QoL domains will be identified, based on patient interviews and the psychometric properties of the existing instruments will be reviewed. Once the instruments have been developed/selected, they will be validated in a pilot study – preferably a Phase II clinical trial – after which the necessary adjustments will be made.

During Phase III, the actual Outcomes Research data will be collected, using the instruments developed during Phase II. At this stage, the randomized clinical trial is the vehicle of choice for data collection because of its high internal validity. However, there are some problems which have to do with the external validity. Randomized clinical trials typically use strict protocols leading to homogeneous patient samples, which may not be representative of the subsequent target population. The generalization of the results may further be complicated by the conditions of patient monitoring and the quality of care, which may not be similar to those in real practice. Nevertheless, despite these apparent limitations, the randomized clinical trial provides the most, if not the only, reliable study design to collect Outcomes Research data on new medicines. When designing a Phase III clinical trial, known to incorporate Outcomes Research parameters, an effort should be made to avoid these difficulties as far as possible. Alternative designs, known as clinical-economic trials or naturalistic prospective economic evaluations have been proposed, with the purpose of making economic evaluations more representative of standard medical practice. These alternative designs may be useful in the post- registration phase, when a new treatment is widely available for use in agreed target patient populations.

References

1 Cartwright AC, Mathews BR: International Pharmaceutical Product Registration. Ellis Hoswood Ltd.:1994.

2 Antiplatelet Trialists' Collaboration: Collaborative overview of randomized trials of antiplatelet treatment. Part I: Prevention of death, myocardial infarction and stroke prolonged antiplatelet treatment. Br Med J 1994;308:81–106.

3 International Stroke Trial. Stroke 1993;24:1618.

4 Muir KW, Lees KR: Clinical experience with excitatory amino acid antagonist drugs. Stroke 1995;26:503–513.

5 Hantson L, De Weerdt W, De Keyser J, Diener JC, et al: The European Stroke Scale. Stroke 1994;25:2215–2219.

Discussion

P. Koudstaal (Rotterdam, Netherlands): What is your personal view of the 6 hour limit for any new trial? Should we use a wider limit and stratify patients into 0–6, 6–12, 12–18 hours, or what should the limits be?

H.C. Diener (Essen, Germany): I think the 6 hour limit is adequate, at least for a few of the experimental drugs that are now being tested, which have shown efficacy in this time period in animal experiments. But I would propose to include in Phase III trials patients who come in up to 12 hours, and stratify accordingly. Perhaps we would have to increase the sample size.

C. Warlow (Edinburgh, Scotland): The problem of trying to find an outcome event for Phase III trials which we can all agree about is very important. Perhaps we could have some sort of hierarchy. We all agree about mortality. We should then think of the next most simple thing, which I suggest relates to the question 'are you dependent on others for day-to-day activities?' Then one could have measures which were a little more complicated. But at least for meta- analyses we should have death and some measure of dependency which is simple and understandable by us all.

H.C. Diener: I totally agree.

Cerebrovasc Dis 1995;5(suppl 1):16–21

S.M. Davis
A. Donnan

Melbourne Neuroscience Centre,
Royal Melbourne Hospital, Victoria,
Australia

Patients, Centres, Admission Procedures and Non-Randomized Treatments around the World

Key Words
Stroke
Trials
Consent
Therapy
Ambulance

Abstract
There are intensive international efforts to test promising interventional therapies for ischaemic stroke. National differences in accrual, management and consent could impact on international stroke trials. Information was sought from stroke investigators in 20 countries concerning stroke rates and hospitalization, trial centres, arrival times and triage, neurological involvement and stroke units, consent protocols and use of unproven stroke therapies. Except in developing nations, most patients are hospitalized. Neurologists rarely care for stroke patients and there are few stroke units, despite their proven value. Delays in hospital arrival and triage are common. However, in some countries, most patients arrive within acute trial time windows. Surrogate trial consent is generally accepted, but is under threat and will reduce accrual of patients with aphasia and depressed conscious state. Prevalent unproven acute therapies include heparin, aspirin and glycerol. Stroke trials networks could increase accrual and coordination of acute therapy trials.

Although there has been a dramatic decrease in population-based mortality rates from acute stroke around the world, individual mortality and morbidity remain high, underpinning the importance of current international efforts to identify acute stroke therapies. Positive results of controlled trials of thrombolytic and antiplatelet therapy in myocardial infarction in the 1980s were rapidly translated into clinical practice [1]. Well designed trials of sufficient size are being performed to evaluate thrombolytic, neuroprotective and other strategies for acute tissue rescue in ischaemic brain [2].

Initial results of a number of thrombolytic trials are now becoming known, with possible benefits shown in selected patients with acute ischaemic stroke treated within 6 hours of onset using intravenous tPA [3, 4], although negative results are reported from trials using intravenous streptokinase [5, 6]. Some acute stroke trials have been substantially confined to single countries [2, 5, 7]. However, many involve international collaboration [4, 8]. To show small, but significant effects on stroke mortality rather than solely morbidity, very large patient numbers will be needed, similar to the successful acute myocardial infarction therapy protocols [9]. Very large trials can be restricted to one country in those with large populations at risk of stroke, as in the USA and Japan. Additionally, systematic overviews will be needed of results from a num-

S.M. Davis
Director of Neurology and Head of Stroke Service
The Melbourne Neuroscience Centre
Royal Melbourne Hospital
Parkville VIC 3050 (Australia)

1015–9770/95/0057–0016
$8.00/0

ber of national or regional studies, to improve statistical power and to gauge the clinical value of interventional therapies [10].

Stroke is not a homogeneous entity around the world. Intracerebral haemorrhage is more common in Chinese [11] and Japanese populations [12], while intracranial atherosclerosis and small vessel disease are more prevalent in Black and Asian populations [13, 14]. Furthermore in some countries, the proportion of stroke subtypes is changing, notably Japan, where there are declining rates of haemorrhage and increasing numbers of lacunar infarcts and extracranial large-vessel infarcts [15]. Although acute stroke case-mortality rates are generally similar around the world [11, 16–20], there may be some significant variations. Swedish and Swiss case-fatality rates are reported to be lower [21, 22], although this might in fact reflect a referral bias because of their high rates of hospitalization, including milder strokes not admitted in other countries [20].

Therefore, in evaluating international multicentre trial results and in conducting meta-analyses, it should be borne in mind that the pathogenesis and outcomes of cerebral infarction is not internationally uniform. To prepare this overview, we sought information from stroke investigators who have been involved in stroke trials and organization in Australia, Canada, France, Germany, Hong Kong, India, Indonesia, Israel, Italy, Japan, New Zealand, Russia, Singapore, South Africa, Sweden, Switzerland, The Netherlands, the United Kingdom and the United States of America.

Patients and Centres

Around the world, about 80% of acute stroke patients are admitted to hospital, although the proportion is much lower in developing nations such as India, where most patients are treated at home. Hospitalization of acute stroke patients approaches 100% in Sweden [21], Switzerland [22] and Russia. In most countries, only a small proportion of patients are admitted to hospitals involved in clinical stroke trials. However, even in a small territory like Hong Kong, with only 5000 new strokes per year, it has been possible to mount a successful clinical trial [23] because 30% of patients are admitted to hospitals participating in stroke trials. At least one third of patients with acute stroke in Switzerland and Sweden are admitted to hospitals participating in clinical trials. In Australia, with a population of 18 million, 40 urban and some rural centres have been involved in the Australian Streptokinase Trial [7].

Transport, Arrival Time and Accrual of Stroke Trial Patients

Short hospital arrival times are crucial for acute interventional stroke trials, given the postulated brief therapeutic windows. Protracted stroke arrival times are a problem around the world, in large part considered to reflect nihilistic attitudes by patients, carers and primary care practitioners. In contrast, rapid arrival times after trauma and acute myocardial infarction correlate with the anticipated benefits of early intervention and treatment. Some delays might reflect geographical factors, with large distances to trial centres in some countries. Delays in stroke arrival are seen as a major problem both in first world countries such as the United States, Japan, Germany and Australia, as well as in developing nations such as India and Indonesia (table 1).

In contrast, some small countries or cities with well coordinated emergency medical services have achieved much shorter hospital arrival times for acute stroke patients. In Sweden, about 43% of patients arrive at hospital within 6 hours. In Switzerland, all patients could potentially be admitted to hospital within 1 hour, because of the large number of small, scattered hospitals and an active helicopter service [22]. The median time for arrival of acute stroke patients is only 4 hours in The Netherlands [24]. In New Zealand, 53% of patients in the Auckland region arrive at hospital within four hours, 69% of stroke patients arrive within six hours in the Tel Aviv area of Israel, while in Hong Kong 63% of stroke patients arrive within twelve hours [25].

Even with rapid transportation to hospitals participating in clinical stroke trials, only a small proportion of patients will be trial-eligible. Only 17 out of 222 patients in a Dutch study with cerebral infarction and an admission delay of less than 6 hours would have been eligible for an acute stroke trial [24] and only 5% of patients arriving at MAST-E trial centres within 6 hours fulfilled entry criteria.

Table 1. Countries with short hospital arrival times after stroke

Country	Hospital arrival time
Switzerland	Potential for most by helicopter <1 hour
New Zealand (Auckland)	53% <4 hours
The Netherlands	Median 4 hours
Israel (Tel Aviv)	69% <6 hours
Sweden	43% <6 hours
Hong Kong	63% <12 hours

Stroke arrival times should be facilitated by better collaboration between patients, relatives, primary care doctors, ambulance services and acute hospitals. Accrual for the MAST-E trial was particularly successful in smaller French cities. in the United States, while there is no national plan, each stroke trial and stroke centre has its own enrolment strategies. There are also important variations in perceptions about stroke by referring family doctors in different countries concerning potentially useful drugs, and their willingness to refer patients to trials centres. This underscores the importance of educating and involving family doctors in stroke trials [26].

An optimal approach for acute stroke management would be for the patient, their relative or bystander to directly call an emergency ambulance number, without the inherent delay involved in consulting a personal physician [27].

Speed of Assessment for Stroke Trials

In trial organization, rapid assessment in the Emergency Department and triage of potential trial patients is vital. In virtually all countries involved in stroke trials, there is ready access to emergency CT brain scanning, although this is still very restricted in some countries such as Russia, Indonesia and India. Delays in recognition and communication in Emergency Departments of potential stroke trial patients are generally seen as more common problems (table 2). In Germany and other countries, it is perceived that delays are often due to house doctors who have a low awareness of acute stroke trials. In Tel Aviv, a successful tactic has been to have a neurologist in the Emergency Department, strokes being seen as the first priority. In the United States a suggested strategy has been to enlist emergency room physicians as trial co-investigators, or even to link reimbursement to the interval from stroke onset. In Australia, a triage nurse in the Emergency Department directly pages the stroke trialist concerning all stroke arrivals, bypassing junior doctors.

Table 2. Identified sources of delay in accrual of patients for stroke trials

Non-emergency attitude to stroke by patients and primary care physicians
Poor coordination of emergency transport services
Emergency room and triage delays
Protracted consent procedures; emergence of laws preventing surrogate consent
Small number of stroke units

Management of Acute Stroke and Stroke Units

An important factor in the accrual of trial patients is whether stroke patients are managed acutely or are accessible to stroke physicians or neurologists involved in acute trials. Around the world, internal medicine physicians and geriatricians, with variable interest and expertise in stroke management, manage the great majority of acute stroke patients. In academic centres, early neurological or stroke physician involvement is much more common. There are interesting geographical differences. For example, in Russia, all stroke patients are looked after by neurologists. In the USA, most are cared for by primary care physicians, and this proportion is thought likely to increase with the emphasis being given to managed care plans in the community setting. In the UK, only 5% of neurologists in one survey routinely managed acute stroke patients [28]. Probably reflecting manpower considerations, neurosurgeons are more involved than neurologists in the acute care of stroke in Japan.

Clinical stroke trials would be facilitated by larger numbers of acute stroke units. Despite the many papers [29–32] indicating that both functional outcome and mortality are improved by management of stroke patients in a specialized area by expert staff, the number of stroke units around the world is still very small and chiefly restricted to academic centres where there is stroke interest and expertise. For example, in the UK, only 5% of physicians looking after acute stroke patients have access to a stroke unit [33]. In contrast, non-intensive stroke units and mobile stroke teams have been established in the great majority of hospitals in Sweden [21]. There are only 50–100 stroke units in the United States, but this is likely to markedly increase following the recent recommendations of the Expert Panel on the Management of Acute Stroke, which endorsed the development of acute stroke units as of proven value and a high priority [27].

While effective acute therapies are awaited, it is unclear which specific stroke unit strategies produce the measured benefits. The implementation of managed care plans for stroke patients, more readily administered in a specialized ward, can shorten bed stay and reduce costs [34]. The structure of stroke units varies considerably. Neurological intensive care units are often the model in Germany [35] and France, whereas in Australia and Sweden, stroke units are generally ward areas with expert staffing, but little monitoring equipment. Other stroke units are essentially neurorehabilitation wards rather than acute treatment facilities.

Consent Procedures

Simplified, ethically sound consent procedures are most important for trial enrolment (table 3). The two key issues of relevance to stroke trials are, firstly, the complexity of the consent procedure and secondly, whether surrogate consent is permitted in patients with aphasia or impaired conscious state. The huge disparity between accrual for the ISIS-2 acute myocardial infarction trial in the UK and USA was thought to have reflected the far more complex consent protocol required in the USA [36]. The UK approach is a less formal one than in the USA, allowing far greater discretion by the individual doctor, with the view that excessively detailed consent can be inhumane, impair trial recruitment and, by delaying the discovery of effective treatments, potentially cause many deaths [36].

While virtually all nations require some form of informed consent, most Ethics Committees will allow surrogate consent by spouse or next of kin if the patient cannot provide consent because of dysphasia or depressed conscious state. Post-treatment consent is permitted in France if the patient is unable to consent and the family is not immediately available. In some Asian countries such as Singapore, 'over-lawyering' is discouraged, and discussion and consent by the family is paramount. In Russia, the final decision could be made by the neurologist in charge of the case. In South Africa, the hospital superintendent can give consent if next of kin are unavailable.

In contrast, in Germany and some districts in Italy, only the patient can consent to involvement. Hence, patients with dysphasia or altered conscious state are excluded from acute trials. In the USA, there are differences in legislation between States and policies by individual institutional review boards, but evolving legal policies might well prohibit surrogate consent. Various patient advocacy and guardianship acts, which prohibit surrogate consent, are already in place in some Australian states and are likely in Canada. One American study indicated that such policies could reduce acute trial accruals by one third and particularly affect entry of patients with more severe, and language-impairing strokes [37].

Non-Randomized Acute Stroke Therapies

Of relevance to patient accrual in acute stroke trials are the prevalent non-randomized acute stroke therapies already in use, most of unproven value [27]. There are significant differences in attitudes of both treating specialists and primary care doctors in different countries, which can impact on the organization of international stroke trials [26]. Heparin is the major therapy used in acute stroke, outside of clinical trials, around the world. In most countries, it is frequently used in cardioembolic stroke, progressive or basilar-territory infarction. In the United States [38, 39], 22% of patients with ischaemic stroke were treated with heparin in the first 24 hours, despite their physicians' widespread concerns about both its efficiency and efficacy [39]. In general, haemodilution is rarely used, except in selected patients with acute ischaemia and elevated haematocrit, although is still apparently prevalent in internal medicine departments in Austria and Russia. Glycerol is widely used in Japan in patients with reduced level of consciousness and is also popular in Germany and Italy. Steroids are frequently used in India and Russia. Nimodipine is little used in ischaemic stroke. However, in a UK survey, about a third of consultants used calcium channel antagonists or high-dose steroids in selected patients [33]. Aspirin is frequently used acutely in most countries. A wide variety of unproven therapies appear to be used in Russia and India.

Table 3. Variations in trial consent procedures around the world

Country	Consent procedure
Most countries	Surrogate consent permitted (next of kin, spouse)
Germany, some districts Italy, some states USA	Only patient can consent
Some Australian states, Canada, some states USA	Various patient advocacy and guardianship acts preventing surrogate consent
Asian countries	Emphasis on consent by family
UK	Less formal consent procedure than in USA with greater discretion by managing doctor
France	Post-treatment consent allowed if patient unable and family unavailable

Stroke Trials Networks

National clinical trials networks are well established in many countries and have facilitated controlled trials in AIDS and cancer. Given the plethora of proposed clinical stroke trials and the array of sponsoring companies, a number of countries have attempted to devise a national strategy for stroke trials, based on a network of accredited centres with expertise to participate in high quality clinical research trials. Formal networks have been set up in Canada (Canadian Stroke Consortium), and in Australia and New Zealand (Australasian Stroke Trials Network). The National Stroke Association in the USA is involved in the organization of sites for collaborative treatment trials, a German Stroke Foundation supports German trials and a Cerebrovascular Disease Study Group has been set up in Italy. In other countries, networks have been assembled for large trials, such as the MAST streptokinase trials in France and Italy, the Dutch TIA trial and the European Cooperative Acute Stroke Study (ECASS). Given the competing demands of different companies and the need for prioritization of trials based on scientific merit as well as infrastructure support, national coordination of stroke trial research seems appropriate. A further development of this concept would be the development of an International Stroke Trials Network, with accreditation of stroke trial centres around the world and coordination between national stroke trial networks.

Acknowledgements

We wish to acknowledge the valuable contributions of our expert colleagues in: Canada (John Norris, Toronto), France (Marc Hommel, Grenoble), Germany (Werner Hacke, Heidelberg), Hong Kong (Richard Kay, Shatin), India (Nadir Bharucha, Bombay), Indonesia (Dede Gunawan, Bandung), Israel (Natan Bornstein, Tel Aviv), Italy (Livia Candelise, Milan), Japan (Takenori Yamaguchi, Osaka), New Zealand (Neil Anderson, Auckland), Russia (Nicolay Yakhno, Moscow), Singapore (Wong Meng Cheong), South Africa (Jacques Joubert, formerly in Pretoria; Vivien Fritz, Johannesburg), Sweden (Bo Norrving, Lund), Switzerland (Julien Bogousslavsky, Lausanne), The Netherlands (Peter Koudstaal, Rotterdam), United Kingdom (Peter Sandercock, Edinburgh), United States of America (Harold Adams, Iowa City).

References

1 Collins R, Julian D: British Heart Foundation surveys (1987 and 1989) of United Kingdom treatment policies for acute myocardial infarction. Br Heart J 1991;66:250–255.
2 Anonymous: Major ongoing stroke trials. Stroke 1995;26:349–353.
3 Yamaguchi T, Hayakawa T, Kiuchi H: The Japanese Thrombolysis Study Group. Intravenous tissue plasminogen activator ameliorates the outcome of hyperacute embolic stroke. Cerebrovasc Dis 1993;3:269–272.
4 Hacke W, Kaste M, Fieschi C: The ECASS Study Group. The efficacy of IV-rtPA in acute ischemic stroke: first results of the ECASS trial [abstract]. Stroke 1995;26:167.
5 Hommel M, Boissel JP, Cornu C, Boutitie F, et al: The MAST Study Group. Termination of trial of streptokinase in severe acute ischaemic stroke [letter]. Lancet 1994;345:57.
6 Donnan GA, Davis SM, Chambers BR, Gates PC, et al: Australian Streptokinase Trial [letter]. Lancet 1995;345:578–579.
7 Donnan GA, Davis SM, Chambers BR, et al: Australian Streptokinase Trial (ASK). In: Del Zoppo GJ, Mori E, Hacke W, eds. Thrombolytic Therapy in Acute Ischemic Stroke II. Berlin: Springer-Verlag, 1993;80–85.
8 Sandercock P: The International Stroke Trial Collaborative Group. International Stroke Trial (IST): Two week mortality in different categories of patients [abstract]. Cerebrovasc Dis 1994;4:221.
9 Sandercock P, Willems H: Medical treatment of acute ischaemic stroke. Lancet 1992;339: 537–539.
10 Counsell C, Warlow C, Sandercock P, Fraser H, Van Gijn J: The Cochrane Collaboration Stroke Review Group. Meeting the need for systematic reviews in stroke care. Stroke 1995; 26:498–502.
11 Kay R, Woo J, Kreel L, Wong HY, Teoh R, Nicholls MG: Stroke subtypes among Chinese living in Hong Kong: The Shatin Stroke Registry. Neurology 1992;42:985–987.
12 Suzuki K, Kutsuzawa T, Takita K, Ito M, et al: Clinico-epidemiologic study of stroke in Akita, Japan. Stroke 1987;18:402–406.
13 Caplan LR, Gorelick PB, Hier DB: Race, sex and occlusive cerebrovascular disease: a review. Stroke 1986;17:648–655.
14 Feldmann E, Daneault N, Kwan E, Ho KJ, Pessin MS, Langenberg, P, Caplan LR: Chinese-white differences in the distribution of occlusive cerebrovascular disease. Neurology 1990; 40:1541–1545.
15 Yamaguchi T, Oita J: Stroke management around the world – Japan. Cerebrovasc Dis 1994;4:437–440.
16 Bonita R, Anderson CS, Broad JB, Jamrozik KD, Stewart-Wynne EG, Anderson NE: Stroke incidence and case fatality in Australasia. A comparison of the Auckland and Perth population-based stroke registers. Stroke 1994;25: 552–557.
17 Bamford J, Sandercock P, Dennis M, Burn J, Warlow C: Classification and natural history of clinically identifiable subtypes of cerebral infarction. Lancet 1991;337:1521–1526.
18 Bamford J, Sandercock P, Dennis M, Burn J, Warlow C: A prospective study of acute cerebrovascular disease in the community: the Oxfordshire Community Stroke Project – 1981–1986. 2. Incidence, case fatality rates and overall outcome at one year of cerebral infarction, primary intracerebral and subarachnoid haemorrhage. J Neurol Neurosurg Psychiatry 1990; 53:16–22.
19 Herman B, Leyten ACM, van Luijk JH, Frenken CWGM, Op de Coul AAW, Schulte BPM: Epidemiology of stroke in Tilburg, The Netherlands. The population-based stroke incidence register: 2. Incidence, initial clinical picture and medical care, and three-week case fatality. Stroke 1982;13:629–634.
20 Norris JW: Stroke management around the world. Cerebrovasc Dis 1994;4:430–440.
21 Asplund K, Webster PO: Stroke management around the world – Sweden. Cerebrovasc Dis 1994;4:432–434.
22 Bogousslavsky J: Stroke management around the world – Switzerland. Cerebrovasc Disc 1994;4:431–432.
23 Kay R, Wong KS, Woo J: Pilot study of low-molecular-weight heparin in the treatment of acute ischemic stroke. Stroke 1994;25:684–685.

24 Herderscheê D, Limburg M, Hijdra A, Bollen A, Pluvier J, te Water W: Timing of hospital admission in a prospective series of stroke patients. Cerebrovasc Dis 1991;1:165–167.
25 Kay R, Woo J, Poon WS: Hospital arrival time after onset of stroke. J Neurol Neurosurg Psychiatry 1992;55:973–974.
26 Kappelle LJ, Adams HP Jr, Torner JC, Bendixen BH: Physician attitudes towards acute stroke – a comparison of primary care physicians in Iowa and The Netherlands. Cerebrovasc Dis 1993;3:364–369.
27 Adams JP Jr, Brott TG, Crowell RM, Furlan AJ, et al: Guidelines for the management of patients with acute ischemic stroke. A statement for healthcare professionals from a special writing group of the Stroke Council, American Heart Association. Stroke 1994;25:1901–1914.
28 Lindley RI, Amayo EO, Marshall J, Sandercock PAG, Dennis M, Warlow CP: The Stroke Association survey of the hospital care of patients with acute stroke in the UK: (1) Hospital organisation and services. Unpublished communication, 1994.
29 Strand T, Asplund K, Eriksson S, Hagg E, Lithner F, Wester PO: A non-intensive stroke unit reduces functional disability and the need for long-term hospitalization. Stroke 1985;16:29–34.
30 Strand T, Asplund K, Eriksson S, Hägg E, Lithner F, Wester PO: Stroke unit care – who benefits? Comparisons with general medical care in relation to prognostic indicators on admission. Stroke 1986;17:377–381.
31 Indredavik B, Bakke F, Solberg R, Rokseth R, Haaheim LL, Holme I: Benefit of a stroke unit: a randomized controlled trial. Stroke 1991;22:1026–1031.
32 Langhorne P, Williams BO, Gilchrist W, Howie K: Do stroke units save lives? Lancet 1993; 342:395–398.
33 Lindley RI, Amayo EO, Marshall J, Sandercock PAG, Dennis M, Warlow CP: The Stroke Association survey of the hospital care of patients with acute stroke in the UK: (2) Immediate medical treatment. Unpublished communication, 1994.
34 Bowen J, Yaste C: Effect of a stroke protocol on hospital costs of stroke patients. Neurology 1994;44:1961–1964.
35 Hacke W, Schwab S, de Georgia M: Intensive care of acute ischemic stroke. Cerebrovasc Disc 1994;4:385–392.
36 Collins R, Doll R, Peto R: Ethics of clinical trials. In: Williams CJ, ed. Introducing New Treatments for Cancer: Practical, Ethical and Legal Problems. Chichester: John Wiley & Sons Ltd, 1992:49–65.
37 Saver JL, Starkman S, Fox S, Saver RS, Biller J: The impact upon clinical stroke trials of restricting informed consent [abstract]. Stroke 1995;26:157.
38 Sanderson DC: How twin cities neurologists treat ischemic stroke. Policies and trends. Arch Neurol 1993;50:1098–1103.
39 Marsh EE III, Adams HP Jr, Biller J, Wasek P, Banwart K, Mitchell V, Woolson R: Use of antithrombotic drugs in the treatment of acute ischemic stroke: a survey of neurologists in practice in the United States. Neurology 1989; 39:1631–1634.

Discussion

K. Prasad (New Delhi, India): I would add to the list of countries where intracerebral haemorrhage is frequent. India is one of them. In a recently concluded analysis of 708 patients consecutively admitted in our hospital with CT scan done in 90% of cases, we found at least one third overall had intracerebral haemorrhage. Between the age group of 41–50 years, 40% had intracerebral haemorrhage. The second point is that for a developing country as a whole there are far more delays in admissions as well as a smaller proportion of patients with acute stroke being admitted. But there is wide variation within the country. In big cities you will find that stroke admissions are as frequent as in any developed country.

S.M. Davis (Melbourne, Australia): The experience in Australia is that often rural centres are very good in accruing patients for stroke trials because patients rapidly get into hospital. Urban centres perhaps have more infrastructure, but rural centres can be very valuable in stroke trials. I believe that in France with MAST-E that was the experience.

B. Ringlestein (Münster, Germany): You addressed the problem of treatment of stroke patients by internal physicians rather than neurologists. One of the reasons for the success of treatment of acute myocardial infarction was that nobody questioned the competence of cardiologists to perform it. However, the competence of neurologists to treat stroke is questioned all over the world for financial among other reasons. What kind of strategy should we face for the future?

S.M. Davis: The treatment of strokes should not be restricted to neurologists. Internal physicians with expertise in stroke should be also involved. I believe that neurologists have been very slow in getting involved. In most countries neurologists have only recently been involved in acute stroke management. I think that stroke units should be developed as a priority in every hospital treating stroke. They could be run by a neurologist or a physician with a particular interest in stroke. The incorporation of critical paths for stroke, managing stroke patients in a special area, will allow us more rapidly to introduce therapies that have been proven to be effective.

Cerebrovasc Dis 1995;5(suppl 1):22–26

J. van Gijn

University Department of Neurology,
Utrecht, The Netherlands

Who Is in Charge? Investigator and Sponsor Alliances

Key Words
Acute stroke trials
Collaboration
Outcome measures
Remuneration
Sponsorship

Abstract
Collaboration between clinical trial investigators and their sponsors must pay attention to certain guidelines if clinical standards are to be maintained and the interests of the patient safeguarded. At issue are questions of remuneration, record-keeping and competence as well as outcome measures and *post-hoc* trial analysis. It is suggested that remuneration for clinical trial involvement should not be set at such a high level that other aspects of patient care may be jeopardized. Trials should be conducted in recognised centres involving experienced trialists with the accuracy of patient records monitored by random audits. The design, data collection and analysis should be the responsibility of a Steering Committee which represents all trial participants. The primary outcome measures in acute stroke trials should assess degree of disability or handicap and surrogate end-points should be treated with caution. The use of sub-group analysis should be limited and any such sub-groups should be defined before the trial commences.

If drug companies had existed in Hippocrates' time, the doctor's oath he drew up would certainly have referred to the need to protect the interests of individual patients as well as of medical science against the pressure of the market. Even in these times, where our own hospital managers now communicate in capitalistic Healthspeak ('providers', 'purchasers', 'production'), physicians should closely safeguard their integrity against immoral attractions of weak study protocols and dubious drug companies. The sins may not always pertain to the deepest pits of corruption and include petty imprecisions but sins they are, incompatible not only with the rules of society but also with the trust specifically placed in doctors by their patients and by the scientific community.

I am no champion of state-controlled economies, not even in the field of drug research. After all, the huge sociological experiment conducted in Eastern Europe and broken off in 1989, 72 years after its inception, has not yielded a single biochemical compound that is a useful addition to our present pharmacopoeia. Commercial profit is not dishonourable in itself, only it is an objective that, if not contained, inevitably conflicts with the more fundamental interests of patients and of the profession. It is that I wish to make a plea for a body of solid rules that help doctors to protect these fundamental interests. This is no blind idealism. Physicians have also managed to draw up rules for organ donation from brain-dead patients. These rules reconcile the commendable aim of providing new organs for handicapped or moribund recipients on the one hand, and the even more fundamental rights of the potential donors on the other. Given that commercial interests are the engine of our society, it should be possible for the medical profession to agree on rules that reconcile these with the interests of science.

J. van Gijn
University Hospital
Box 85500
3508 GA Utrecht (The Netherlands)

1015–9770/95/0057–0022
$8.00/0

Clinician and Investigator and Fund Raiser?

It is difficult enough for the physician to combine the role of carer and scientist. Patients entrust their health problems to general practitioners and specialists in the hope of obtaining a cure, and with the knowledge that there are diseases for which there is no cure, but mostly they are not prepared for the 'perhaps's' and 'maybe's' of a clinical trial protocol. Not infrequently the procedure of 'informed consent' gives patients the impression that the doctors are primarily serving their own ends rather than those of their patients. The well-known phraseology that 'we wish you to have the best treatment in the world but in your case and at this point nobody really knows what the best treatment is' does not leave every patient with an unshaken belief in the hospital's competence. At any rate patients often forget about the actual purpose of the trial, or even about whether they were free in their decision to participate [1, 2]. This may become less of a problem with increasing public awareness of the importance of clinical trials: ideally patients should start wondering why they are not asked to participate in a clinical trial rather than the reverse. Yet it is more realistic to expect that this will remain a delicate conversation. Fortunate is the physician whose motives are unselfish and purely consist of the will to improve the body of medical knowledge, and thereby to improve the chances of recovery for future patients. Personal ambition may be a factor, but in most trials this factor is diluted by the participation of many other physicians.

Motives become more questionable when remuneration becomes a factor. Things are hardly made easier if the money does not go to the doctor's own pocket but to the department research fund, as is often the case. The success of a clinical department, particularly in a university hospital, is intricately linked with tangible and intangible gains of the persons involved: tenure, promotion, and the esteem of one's colleagues. In those cases an impartial outsider might wonder whether the attempt to obtain the patient's consent is really as dispassionate and harmless as it should be. The question is not whether there should be any remuneration at all, but whether this exceed the payment for other activities.

Over-Payment is Unethical

Money is at the root of all evil, and clinical trials are no exception. Of course it is quite in order for pharmaceutical firms to reimburse clinicians for the time they invest and the expenses they make in entering patients in the trial. The problem arises only when entering patients into a sponsored trial is much more profitable per unit of time than seeing patients in the clinic – or entering patients into a non-commercial trial! Regrettable though it is, current medical practice is still replete with treatment regimens inherited from the pre-trial era, and current generations have to work their way through a backlog of trials that would have been done decades ago if the appropriate methodology and insight had been available. Examples of such 'catching-up trials' are the benefits of carotid endarterectomy [3], or of anticoagulant treatment in patients with atrial fibrillation and a TIA or non-disabling ischaemic stroke [4]. Other trials that need to be done but are uninteresting from a commercial point of view are those with old drugs for new indications, such as aspirin in the secondary prevention of important vascular events [5].

The choice of clinicians about which clinical trials they wish to join should be motivated not by worries about where to find next year's salaries for their data managers or trusted colleagues, or about how to create a fund for carrying out the type of research they really want to do. Rather such decisions should have to do with how burning is the issue under investigation, from the perspective of health care, science, or both.

The Need for Quality Control

In the US, the Food and Drug Administration (FDA) performs routine checks on clinical investigators of new drugs. In the course of these regulatory checks some appalling examples of scientific misconduct were uncovered. An obstetrician gave false information about having used a particular analgesic during delivery; a psychiatrist with a good reputation for his prompt reporting of the results of antidepressants was found in a completely empty office; a rheumatologist supplied faked laboratory results; a neurologist was found to have submitted identical reports about patients with Parkinson's disease in two different studies, with two different sponsors, and a cardiologist involved in a study of a drug for treating congestive heart failure changed the radiologist's report about chest X-rays so that the drug would seem more effective [6]. This list of forgeries is far from exhaustive, and can be supplemented with a multitude of instances in which investigators were not outright dishonest but definitely careless.

It is a disturbing thought that in Europe most national licensing bodies have taken a rather cavalier attitude towards the conduct of clinical investigations. Criticisms may be directed at the interpretation of trial results. The results themselves are often accepted on trust, even if the potential market for the new drug in question is vast, with huge amounts of money at stake. Things are now on the mend, because the European Community has recently formulated guidelines for the conduct of clinical trials ('Good Clinical Practice'), with strong recommendations to have these adopted by the member states. These rules include not only requirements for the design of clinical studies but also for auditing of case record forms. Yet it will be some time before all European countries have reached the level of quality control that is customary in the US. It is honourable but naive to have too much faith in people's conscience when the enticements are so great. On the other hand, clinicians should not be buried in paperwork. Auditing of random samples rather than of every single case record form seems a reasonable compromise.

Trial Participants Should Have a Good Track Record - and Companies too

Money may not stink, but some trials do. Everybody knows examples of clinical trials with new drugs of which many do not really trust the results. Such examples exist also in the field of acute stroke, or in the secondary prevention of stroke. Not only have these studies been conducted without the close monitoring by an independent body that is customary in the US. One also observes close and rather exclusive links between the industry in question and a small number of hospitals, none of which is or has been active in other areas of stroke research.

For trial results to be acceptable to the scientific community, short of the rigid rules applied in the US, one of the requirements is that the centres involved have proved capable of good clinical research in the field, also in types of research that do not depend on industrial sponsoring. In other words, pharmaceutical companies would be wise in choosing hospital groups that have earned themselves a good name in medical science, on the basis of regular publications in peer-reviewed journals.

Similarly, clinicians should beware of pharmaceutical companies that in the past have earned licenses by means of small trials, conducted in small centres. Of course drug companies may better their lives but if the track record is not very good there is even more reason than usual for making water-tight arrangements about the protocol and the conduct of the trial (see below). Also, drug companies embarking on clinical trials should have these registered at some central office, with the obligation to report the results – even if they are disappointing.

Measures of Outcome – a Useful Litmus Test

The problem of how to choose the best measure of outcome in a trial is one of the greatest stumbling blocks in trials of acute stroke and deserves a treatise in itself [7]. Traditionally, so-called 'stroke scales' have been applied for this aim, analogous to scales for other neurological conditions such as Parkinson's disease or multiple sclerosis. Although the stated purpose of 'stroke scales' is to measure outcome, these scales are nothing but codifications of the neurological examination, developed for no other purpose than that of localizing lesions within the nervous system. With such a diagnostic approach different functions of the nervous system are separately assessed: power of limbs, speech, visual fields, etc. This reductionist, mechanistic notion of brain function reflects the localisationists' position in the scientific battle that raged in the second half of the 19th century, the opposing party being that of equipotentiality. A brief note about this part of neurological history is therefore in order.

The equipotentialists believed that the brain worked as a unitary system, brain tissue being omnipotent and flexible in its function. Consequently, brain damage would result in a decrease in the overall level of performance, not in a loss of specific functions. The champion of the equipotentialists was the French physiologist Flourens, who supported his views with experiments on dogs and pigeons, in the 1820s. The opposing concept, that of localisation of specific functions, was propounded in a somewhat bizarre fashion by the anatomists Gall and Spurzheim, in a series of books published between 1810 and 1819. They believed that every intellectual and moral property had its own position on the surface of the brain, and that the degree of development of these dispositions could be identified by locating overlying protuberances on the skull. Despite these eccentricities, the theory of localisation gained respectability after the stimulation experiments of Fritsch and Hitzig on anaesthetized dogs, published in 1870, in which they found that weak electrical currents applied through platinum electrodes to the anterior regions of the brain surface produced muscle contractions in the opposite half of the body. The clash between the adherents of the two theories culminated in 1881, at the Third International Congress of Medicine held in London [8]. The equipotentialists were represented by the German physiologist Goltz, who showed the audience a dog in which substantial portion of the brain had been removed by means of a water hose. Yet the animal could still move all limbs, trunk and tail, and had retained all his senses. Later it would turn out that the lesions were less extensive than had been claimed, and on the same afternoon Ferrier showed two chimpanzees, one completely deaf after removal of the auditory cortex, the other limping with a hemiplegic gait after extirpation of the contralateral motor area (the sight of which led Charcot to exclaim: 'Mais c'est un patient!').

The localisationists had won the day, but they had won too completely. The greater part of the brain has no 'primary' motor, sensory, or cognitive tasks, and serves to connect and integrate the separate 'functions'. Similarly, everyday life consists of a multitude of tasks that are integrated and difficult to separate. Mood, initiative and speed of thinking are some of the essential features of human life that can be severely affected by stroke but are sadly ignored in 'stroke scales'. It is therefore naive to try and rebuild an entire human being from separate 'functions' as if it were a jigsaw puzzle, even apart from the insoluble problem of how to weight and add up the different items to something meaningful. A patient is more than the sum of his signs [9]. For clinical trials aimed at testing drugs in 'real life' (Phase III trials) a higher, more integrated level of measurement is needed, that is, scales should measure function not at the level of the organ (impairments) but at the level of the person (disability scales), or even at the level of social interaction (handicap scales) [10]. What really counts for patients is what they can do in life, compared with what they want to do, or were once able to do.

Many pharmaceutical industries are fond of outcome measures at a low level of integration, because these, though of little relevance, are 'objective', can be quantified and even with small trials lend themselves to statistical massage from which some kind of p values emerge. Not all licensing bodies are equally quick in perceiving how completely meaningless these calculations are. In many Western countries drugs have been licensed merely on the basis of effects on specific functions, or with even more flimsy evidence, of effects on MRI scans, laboratory animals, or cell cultures. In fact such 'proxy outcome events' are acceptable only in preliminary stages of research (Phase II trials), to explore whether there is a biological effect at all. For application in regular practice, the FDA has now firmly and sensibly taken the position that new drugs for neurological diseases are allowed only if an effect on disability has been demonstrated.

Who is in Charge?

Sponsors derive certain rights from their investments, but this does not include the right to exclude clinicians from essential activities to do with the quality and credibility of the trial. Drawing up the protocol, storing the data, planning interim analyses, and prior definition of subgroups are grave responsibilities that should be shared between sponsor and participants. This shared commitment should be reflected in the formation of a single Steering Committee as the highest authority of the study, in which all parties are represented. The selection of clinicians in the Steering Committee should be made by the participants, and not by the sponsor.

In this day and age it is unacceptable for responsible clinicians to be confronted by changes in the protocol or interim analyses which have been initiated entirely by the industry in question, without involvement of a Steering Committee in which the participating physicians are represented. Similarly, trial forms should be sent for checking and inclusion in the data base not to the company in question, but to an independent office, run under the direction of one of the clinical participants or of an epidemiologist – provided the people involved have a good track record in unsponsored research. It has been rightly argued that the group responsible for data collection and analysis should be financially independent from the results of the trial [11].

Subgroup analyses, if any, should be planned in advance. No doubt most participants in the trial that compared ticlopidine and aspirin in the secondary prevention of stroke (TASS study) feel embarrassed by ludicrous attempts at inflating the tiny and non-significant advantage for ticlopidine by means of a plethora of subgroup analyses: diabetics, patients with TIAs rather than strokes, blacks, and elderly [12].

Conclusions

Cooperation between pharmaceutical industries and physicians is necessary and desirable, but because the parties have different objectives the quality of sponsored studies should be safeguarded by a set of rules, which should at least include the following:

1. Remuneration should not exceed that for other activities, such as patient care or clinical trials commissioned by governments. Reconciling the duties of patient care with those of science is difficult enough without the added bias of having to keep the department alive.

2. Accuracy of patient records should be monitored at the least by means of random audits.
3. Participants in a sponsored trial should have been active in other, non-sponsored clinical research to be credible.
4. Pharmaceutical firms should preferably have a good track record of open cooperation with experienced trialists.
5. The primary measure of outcome in a trial of acute stroke should be the degree of disability or handicap. Surrogate end points in terms of specific impairments or investigations are credible only in the context of a preliminary study that leads up to a proper trial; they can never form the basis for introduction of a drug into routine clinical practice.
6. Definitive formulation of the protocol, collection of data, and analysis should be performed under the responsibility of a Steering Committee, in which the participants are duly represented.
7. Subgroup analysis should be sparse and planned in advance.

Acknowledgement

A. Algra, MD, gave expert comments on an earlier draft of the manuscript.

References

1 Oddens BJ, Algra A, Van Gijn J: [How much information is retained by participants in clinical trials?] Hoe goed zijn deelnemers aan een klinisch onderzoek geinformeerd? Ned Tijdschr Geneeskd 1992;136:2272–2276.
2 Oddens BJ, Algra A, Van Gijn J: Informing patients about clinical trials. Clin Invest 1993; 71:572–573.
3 European Carotid Surgery Trialists' Collaborative Group. MRC European Carotid Surgery Trial: interim results for symptomatic patients with severe (70–99%) or with mild (0–29%) carotid stenosis. Lancet 1991;337:1235–1243.
4 EAFT (European Atrial Fibrillation Trial) Study Group: Secondary prevention in nonrheumatic atrial fibrillation after transient ischaemic attack or minor stroke. Lancet 1993;342: 1255–1262.
5 Antiplatelet Trialists' Collaboration: Collaborative overview of randomised trials of antiplatelet therapy – I: Prevention of death, myocardial infarction, and stroke by prolonged antiplatelet therapy in various categories of patients. Br Med J 1994;308:81–106.
6 Kohn A: False Prophets – Fraud and Error in Science and Medicine. Oxford: Basil Blackwell; 1986.
7 Van Gijn J: Measurement of outcome in stroke prevention trials. Cerebrovasc Dis 1992;2 (suppl 1):23–34.
8 Thorwald J: Das Weltreich der Chirurgen. Stuttgart: Steingrüben;1957.
9 Van Gijn J, Warlow CP: Down with stroke scales! Cerebrovasc Dis 1992;2:244–246.
10 Wood PNH, Badley EM: People with disabilities: toward acquiring information which reflects more sensitively their problems and needs. New York: World Rehabilitation Fund; 1980.
11 Bogousslavsky J: Acute stroke trials: from morass to Nirvana? Cerebrovasc Dis 1959;5:3–6.
12 Van Gijn J, Algra A: Ticlopidine, trials, and torture. Stroke 1994;25:1097–1098.

Discussion

B. Musch (Belgium): As a physician working in a pharmaceutical company, we have to work on the basis of the same ethical principles that guide the work of all physicians. With 20 years of personal experience in this field I think that nowadays the companies that are involved in indications like stroke are looking for efficient and useful ways of interacting with investigators. Ultimately there may be different ways of approaching the programme but our objectives and aims are the same as the objectives and aims of other scientists, which is to find a new drug for our patients. I do not see any value in opposition between the industry and other physicians because I think that we are working towards the same objective and aims.

J. van Gijn (Utrecht, The Netherlands): I made my talk a bit provocative. But there is no denying that there are nuances. I think that there are many examples of problems in society in general, and in medicine in particular caused by different perspectives. But there also many examples of how these different aims have been reconciled by making a good set of rules and that is what we should do.

Cerebrovasc Dis 1995;5(suppl 1):27–30

J. Grotta

Department of Neurology,
University of Texas, USA

A Glimpse to the Future: Multitherapy Trials

Key Words
Acute stroke treatment
Ischaemic cascade
Multimodal therapy
Neuroprotection
Reperfusion

Abstract
Multi-modality therapy for acute ischaemic stroke is an emerging concept stimulated by the existing vacuum in stroke treatment and an increasing understanding of the ischaemic cascade. Experimental studies have shown that infarct size can be reduced more by combinations of reperfusion and neuroprotective strategies than by either one alone. An optimal combination regimen remains to be determined, but will probably target several sequential events occurring after ischaemia. Many logistic hurdles must be overcome before multimodality therapy can be properly tested in clinical trials. This will require a combination of pragmatism, adherence to scientific principles, and international cooperation among clinic investigators.

Most clinical researchers in the stroke field adhere to the concept that the best (most effective) treatment for acute ischaemic stroke will be some combination of therapies. At one time this belief could be supported only by logic and successes in other organ systems, most notably the heart. However, experimental work over the last 15 years in cell culture and animal stroke models has documented the now well recognized 'ischaemic cascade' of sequential events following an abrupt cessation of blood flow subsequently leading to neuronal death. One consequence of this understanding is the targeting of multiple steps along this cascade for therapeutic intervention.

The Ischaemic Cascade

Several variables exist which may effect the ischaemic cascade and consequently the severity of stroke, most importantly the depth of blood flow reduction, its duration before reperfusion occurs, its distribution (i.e., global or focal), and the adequacy of reperfusion assuming it does occur. However, many of the events that have been described seem to follow in a fairly predictable order.

First there is reduction of blood flow followed rapidly by inhibition of protein synthesis, depletion of intracellular energy stores, membrane depolarization, and release of extracellular potassium. This is accompanied by an initial increase in oxygen extraction and glucose metabolism, and lactic acidosis. Membrane depolarization causes opening of voltage operated calcium channels allowing disruption of tightly regulated neuronal calcium homeostasis. Glutamate is released from presynaptic stores, and in the presence of glycine activates the NMDA receptor. The immediate consequence is increased sodium permeability and cellular swelling, but the more damaging event is further elevation of intracellular calcium through the NMDA associated ion channel. Further perturbations in ion flux occur as a result of glutamate's effect on the

J. Grotta
University of Texas
Department of Neurology
6431 Fannin Street
Houston, Texas (USA)

1015–9770/95/0057–0027
$8.00/0

AMPA and metabotropic receptors. Documented increases in other neurotransmitters such as GABA, dopamine, and norepinephrine may also be damaging.

Increased intracellular calcium activates a large number of damaging enzymatic pathways. Calcium (through calmodulin) activates protein kinases such as Cam-kinase II and protein kinase C which may imbalance neuronal homeostasis by causing protein phosphorylation. Other pivotal enzyme systems activated by calcium include the proteases such as calpain which causes cytoskeletal proteolysis, lipases such as phospholipase A which leads to production of arachidonic acid and free radical formation and phospholipase C which results in release of intracellular calcium stores, and nitric oxide synthase resulting in increased damaging NO.

Sequential Effects

Increased gene expression in ischaemic regions, possibly induced by spreading depolarizations after ischaemia, has many damaging consequences. Cytokines such as TNF and IL-1 result in tissue inflammation, and adhesion molecules such as ICAM-1 result in white blood cell interaction with vascular endothelium to produce blood brain barrier damage and may also plug up the microcirculation resulting in 'no reflow'. Growth factors such as NGF and BDNF may result in increased production of NO and also have been reported to be protective when exogenously administered.

While this summary is only a cursory overview of documented neurochemical changes after ischaemia, a therapy targeting only one of these processes is unlikely to result in a therapeutic 'home run' (or 'world cup'). I would make the analogy that these events are like the 'invading hordes'; stop only the first wave and the reinforcements in the subsequent waves will get you; and bombarding the reinforcements without turning back the first attack will also do no good. Carrying this analogy further at the risk of oversimplification to make my point, reduction of CBF can be equated with the first wave, release of neurotransmitters the second, calcium entry the third, enzyme activation the fourth, NO and free radical production the fifth, gene expression the sixth, microvascular/WBC adhesion the seventh, and apoptosis the eighth. Reperfusion strategies are directed at the first wave and various 'neuroprotective' strategies at the second through eighth.

Reperfusion Plus Neuroprotection

Experimental evidence supports the concept that establishing reperfusion alone is not enough. We have shown that reduction of CBF below 10% of baseline for more than 10 minutes of global or 1 hour of focal ischaemia in rats results in extensive binding of neuronal calmodulin with calcium, and consequent activation and then translocation/inactivation of Cam-kinase II. If CBF is restored to normal after these ischaemic thresholds, calcium homeostasis is not reestablished unless a glutamate receptor or voltage channel blocker is administered during the ischaemic interval [1–3].

Combinations of reperfusion and neuroprotective strategies have been shown to be effective in several laboratories. Uematsu found that neuronal calcium signal increased after MCA occlusion in rats and this was not attenuated by reperfusion. The non-competitive NMDA ion channel blocker MK-801 administered during ischaemia was able to attenuate intracellular calcium and increased the amount of neuronal salvage over that achieved only by reperfusion. The addition of the dihydropyridine voltage operated calcium channel antagonist nimodipine to MK-801 augmented the beneficial effect on both calcium and neuronal necrosis [4].

Zivin found a positive effect of the thrombolytic tPA in a rabbit autologous clot embolism model. While MK-801 had no beneficial effect by itself in this model, when added to tPA it was able to increase efficacy by approximately 33% over that achieved by tPA alone [5].

In our laboratory, we were unable to find any additive effect of combining a voltage operated calcium channel antagonist (nicardipine) to a competitive antagonist of glutamate at the NMDA receptor (CGS-19755). Both were modestly effective alone [6]. This finding has reinforced in our minds the necessity of including an attack on the 'first wave', i.e., reduced CBF, in any combination strategy.

More recently we have studied blood substitutes as reperfusion agents, and combined one of these with a promising neuroprotective drug. DCLHb (diaspirin crossed linked haemoglobin) is derived from human erythrocytes and has the same oxygen dissociation characteristics as normal haemoglobin in human red cells. Therefore, it is an ideal haemodiluting agent; it can be given as an intravenous solution resulting in haemodilution without loss of oxygen carrying capacity. A post ischaemic exchange and top load of DCLHb (lowering rat haematocrit from 50% to 30%) reduced infarct volume and almost doubled the duration of MCA occlusion that could be tolerated before neuronal necrosis began to be seen.

Lubeluzole is a sodium and calcium channel blocker which may have an effect on glutamate induced NO production. We have found that post-ischaemic administration of this drug also reduces infarct volume but does not prolong the duration of MCA occlusion tolerated. The combination of DCLHb and lubeluzole had an additive effect reducing ischaemic damage to less than 33% of that measured in controls, while at the same time prolonging to over 2 hours the duration of MCA occlusion that could be tolerated before any permanent neuronal necrosis was produced.

While the promise of multi-modality therapy for stroke is exciting, the clinical reality is that, to my knowledge, no trials combining two or more therapeutic strategies for acute stroke are either planned or underway. One explanation is that too few experimental laboratories have the resources and desire to evaluate this approach and arrive at an optimal therapeutic 'recipe'. This would require a model that is reproducible and simple enough to compare multiple therapeutic trials over time using a large number of rats. Furthermore, funding would probably have to come from a source with an interest in multi-modality therapy (presumably not a pharmaceutical company). Such experimental work, some of which has been cited above, is just beginning to appear in the literature. A great deal of work exploring different logical (and perhaps illogical) drug combinations needs to be done before committing resources to a clinical trial.

Financial issues are presently an important impediment to multi-modality clinical trials. Presumably, no pharmaceutical sponsor wants their drug approved if it could only be administered with another. Understandably, there is great competition to leave the 'first tracks' in the powder field of acute stroke therapy since the likely rewards (both financial and personal) will be great.

Future Prospects: Expanding Trials

I am optimistic that this problem will be solved soon. In my opinion, once the first drug is found to be effective and approved for treating stroke, there will be a rush to 'add on' additional therapies. This is what is happening in the arena of stroke therapies. This is what is happening in the arena of stroke prevention where various other platelet antiaggregants, lipid lowering drugs, or surgery (carotid endarterectomy) are being added to aspirin and compared with therapy with aspiring alone. There will be several incentives for such an approach in treating acute stroke as there currently are in stroke prevention. First, it will be unethical to withhold a proven effective treatment. New therapies will have to be added on to the proven drug in patients who have been conclusively shown to benefit from it. Furthermore, it may be logistically and statistically easier to demonstrate that a new drug adds something (even a little bit) to an existing treatment than to show that it is beneficial as stand alone therapy.

There may be pressure from pharmaceutical companies simply to compare their new drug to a proven effective one in order to obtain regulatory approval based only on demonstration of an equivalent effect. However, because of the experimental data I have just reviewed, I think we should insist on at least one therapeutic arm testing combined therapy trying to build on the effect of what has already been shown to work.

In the event that the Phase III studies of single modality treatments that are now ongoing are negative, in my opinion we should cease wasting time and resources on these individual approaches and design a rational multimodality trial based on results from animal studies, some of which have been described in this presentation.

Multi-modality trials, while promising greater benefits, will also carry greater costs, in particular the need for many patients to fill several comparative treatment arms. This will require an increased number of clinical centres and clinical researchers, and the evolution of simplified trial design and data recording and analysis. We can see this process already beginning. The present round of thrombolytic and neuroprotective trials are at least national, and often intercontinental in scope. While some centres have more experience and are more organized, accurate, and productive than others, we are all learning in the process how to carry out good research in an extremely challenging clinical arena. As an international consortium of centres evolves from this process, my hope is that scientific knowledge and clinical wisdom be our guide in choosing and testing multiple therapies.

References

1 DeGraba TJ, Ostro PT, Strong RA, Earls RM, Zong EJ, Grotta JC: The temporal relation of calcium – calmodulin binding and neuronal damage after global ischemia. Stroke 1992;23:876–882.
2 DeGraba T, Ostrow P, Grotta J: Threshold of calcium disturbances after focal cerebral ischemia in rats – implications of the window of therapeutic opportunity. Stroke 1993;24:1212–1217.
3 Aronowski J, Waxham N, Grotta J: Neuronal protection and preservation of calcium/ calmodulin-dependent protein kinase II and protein kinase C activity by dextrorphan treatment in global ischemia. J Cereb Blood Flow Metab 1993;13:550–557.
4 Uematsu D, Araki N, Greenberg J, Sladky J, Reivich M: Combined therapy with MK-801 and nimodipine for protection of ischemic brain damage. Neurology 1991;41:88–94.
5 Zivin J, Mazzarella V: Tissue plasminogen activator plus glutamate antagonist improves outcome after embolic stroke. Arch Neurol 1991;48:1235–1238.
6 Grotta JC, Picone CM, Dedman JR, Rhoades HM, Strong RA, Earls RM, Yao LP: Neuronal protection correlates with prevention of calcium-calmodulin binding. Stroke 1990;21 (Suppl III):28–31.

Cerebrovasc Dis 1995;5(suppl 1):31–33

Chairman: *J. Bogousslavsky*

Lausanne, Switzerland

Panel Discussion

J. Bogousslavsky (Lausanne, Switzerland): I would like ask to Dr. Marc Fisher to tell us about the present situation in the United States. Is there such a thing as a consortium; have you developed any networks like those in Canada?

M. Fisher (Massachusetts, USA): First of all I would like to thank you for inviting me to participate in this very interesting and thought provoking Symposium. The answer to your question is that, as far as I know, in the United States there is no official organisation for getting investigators together. We are drawn together by the organizers of the trial which is typically the pharmaceutical industry.

I think that there are two major themes that emerged from what the speakers were presenting. The first I would call 'Who, when, how, and what?' Who do we treat, when do we treat them, how do we treat them, (single versus multi-therapy) and lastly, what are the outcome measures that we should employ? The second point that I would emphasize are issues that were raised about trial organisation. There are many such issues that should be discussed.

J. Bogousslavsky: Dr. Sawada, what about Japan? What are the differences and similarities with what you have heard?

T. Sawada (Osaka, Japan): In Japan, all the problems described today are encountered in the same way. There is no difference between Europe and Japan concerning the development of new drugs. But in the case of acute stroke therapy, there are some extra problems. You asked 'Do we really need acute stroke trials?' The answer in Japan is that we really do. In Japan the expected life-span is now almost 80 years. The current rate of elderly people in the total population is 13% but it will be 26% in the coming 25 years. Within 20 years, the expenditure for strokes in elderly people is expected to amount to more than a half of total national income. We have just estimated the total expenditure for stroke patients for last year. For one stroke patient for five years, we have to pay 10 million Japanese yen. The largest component of the cost is for nursing care. So we have to reduce the total expenditure for stroke care and we have to reduce the disability at the acute stage.

J. Bogousslavsky: We always come back to the measurement of effects which is certainly central to the problem of stroke trials. I would like to ask Professor van Gijn about the problem of quality of life. To some it seems that the concept of quality of life is too subjective to be reliable. If I take the example of a very severe right-sided hemispheral infarct with complete anosognosia, perhaps you would accept that the quality of life for the patient is not so bad, but it is for the other people around him. Do you think that we should stop at the level of disability rather than handicap or quality of life?

J. van Gijn (Utrecht, The Netherlands): I think consideration of quality of life is impractical and perhaps it will always be. If you ask a patient who only has half a brain how happy he is, and he says 'quite happy'. Does that count? That is an almost insuperable problem, philosophical and ethically. But even if you ask people in wheelchairs who have transverse lesions of the spinal cord whether they are happy or not with quality of life instruments, after a couple of years they turn out to be quite happy. If you had a drug that was supposed to cure spinal cord lesions, and people in wheelchairs were happy, you could never find whether the drug works or helps. For the time being, I am content to assess disability with a little bit of handicap thrown in. Quality of life is too difficult now. Perhaps it will be too difficult forever.

1015–9770/95/0057–0031
$8.00/0

L.M. Brass (West Haven, USA): I agree that the quality of life measures for stroke are currently impractical. But I do not think that should stop us from pursuing that line of investigation. The situation may not be as dismal as you portray, because I think there are ways of making it more quantitative. It is also important to be clear whether we are using quality of life to decide whether medication works or whether we should apply it in a given setting. I think that our current goal is first to find effective therapies, and then to decide whether the hemiplegic patient is appropriate for treatment. I also think that changes over time may be very useful. Although the hemiplegic may have a different perception of their quality of life, improvements are detectable with some of the quality of life measures. I hope that at one of these meetings we will be able to present data to show that they perform as well (although with different shortcomings) as the other disability scales.

J. Bogousslavsky: Another point which is also methodological is the need for homogeneous groups of patients to enter the trials, as opposed to the clinical routine. Because we would like to have treatment which is effective also in, say, vertebral strokes, but such patients tend to be specially excluded from trials. How do we think we can reconcile that? Do we think it is simply by increasing the number of patients in trials and then sub-grouping, or is there another possibility?

H.C. Diener (Essen, Germany): I do not see another possibility. It may be necessary to increase the stratification factors, let us say for anterior circulation strokes versus posterior circulation strokes, and define how you make the analysis beforehand. With large numbers, such an approach may show a positive trend or a significant result.

H.J.M. Barnett (Ontario, Canada): There are times with a good data base when looking at the subgroups will lead you to the generation of hypotheses. In the Canadian Aspirin Study we did not find a benefit for women. But it eventually transpired that women do not do as badly when they suffer from ischaemic events as do men. So that subgroup analysis was worthwhile, to find an hypothesis which was then looked at. Subgroups do not lead to treatment, but I think to dismiss them altogether is ridiculous if you have a good database.

J. Bogousslavsky: That is true, but sometimes the subgroups are made after the trial has been completed and this is certainly one of the problems. Do you think that the subgroups should be defined earlier and also perhaps balanced in each arm of the treatment?

H.J.M. Barnett: In 1969 when we planned the Canadian Aspirin Study, no clinical trial in stroke had ever been done. Nobody had ever thought about the difference between men and women. We could not plan it in advance because it was a whole new concept. Women do differ in many drug responses. And now that we know it, we would stratify for them, or include them in the design. But when you are at the beginning of things, you cannot put everything in the design.

J. Bogousslavsky: We are in the dilemma now of treating stroke as a single entity while we know that it consists of many different conditions under the same name.

I would now invite members of the audience to ask questions or make specific comments about what you have heard today.

G. Boysen (Hvidovre, Denmark): With drugs other than aspirin we know that women have a different way of reacting. It may be because of their different metabolism. I would like to advocate that in future trials we not only stratify for posterior circulation strokes, for instance, but that we also stratify between men and women so that we will be able to analyze the effect in women. Otherwise one will hardly ever be able to say anything for sure in women.

M.G. Bousser (France): This applies to the surgery trial, where the risk of surgery is higher in women, and the event rate is lower so that the overall benefit does not exist in women. If I remember correctly, the relative risk reduction in the study was 17% in women compared to 69% in men.

On a different topic, I think we all agree that we need more stroke units. But when we discuss this with our authorities we have to warn them that we need more stroke rehabilitation units and institutions for out-patients, because as our Japanese colleague said, these patients are old people. They are often alone and most of them will not recover sufficiently to be able to go back home. So we do need more stroke clinics, we also say we do need more stroke rehabilitation units and more specialized institutions for these patients. It is useless to care about stroke patients in the first few hours if we do not properly organize what goes on afterwards.

C. Fieschi (Rome, Italy): There is an anti-oxidant agent that has been marketed recently for treating or preventing post sub-arachnoid haemorrhagic brain damage in men. This has been marketed in Denmark, Sweden and Austria, for men only. What should we do? Should we set up a process to intervene in this decision? That might prevent male patients in Denmark, Sweden and Austria from being treated with an effective drug. I think that some freedom of decision and some post-marketing surveillance is even more important than designing very large networks.

Talking of networks, I want to say a word in favour of exploratory trials. Take for instance the ganglioside study that was published recently by Professor Lenzi in which we participated. As a result of his trial, gangliosides were not proposed to be marketed for stroke. This is the result of a multi-centre but exploratory trial. I think that exploratory trials, well conducted and discussed at the scientific level as was done here, bring information that allows us to proceed further without having to wait for much more complicated machinery. Let us try to work honestly and scientifically in smaller groups and in exploratory studies before setting up very large, complicated networks of stroke trialists.

J. Bogousslavsky: On the question of men and women, there are certainly obvious clinical and biological differences in some subgroups. The problem is where to stop in order not to make too many subgroups at the beginning. This is a major problem if you do not want to have trials with the tens of thousands of patients which will be needed in order to have enough in each subgroup.

N. Bornstein (Tel Aviv, Israel): The message that I have heard here is that we should have a large body to decide on which compound we should aim in our large-scale studies. I feel this might be dangerous because in avoiding other compounds such a distinguished panel of investigators might prevent some beneficial drugs from being tested. Perhaps the aim should be to have a committee which should decide on several drugs to be tested and perhaps this committee should also decide on the centres that should participate because, as has been mentioned, some centres are not appropriate for drug trials. We should be open-minded and all drugs should be tested in order to get the right answer.

J.M. Orgogozo (Bordeaux, France): Professor van Gijn said in his conclusion that what is interesting is not assessable, and what is assessable is not interesting. I think that is not entirely true. Among the interesting domains, that is quality of life and handicap, there is a way to analyse the components which are sometimes dismissed as not interesting. One example of this new approach is eligibility for benefit which is often forgotten. If you look at the link between quality of life and handicap, you find that in some countries like France, patients who are more handicapped have a better quality of life because they reach the threshold of eligibility for benefit. And these are aspects that we can measure. So I make a plea not to be nihilistic in the domains of assessment of stroke outcome, but to use the components of impairment and disability as elements to understand and measure the higher order dimensions.

P. Koudstaal

Rotterdam, The Netherlands

Closing Remarks

On behalf of Professor Bogousslavsky and my co-chairman Professor Barnett, I would like to end this interesting Symposium by thanking all the speakers for their excellent presentations. They have taken us through the problems of acute stroke trials, the problems of organisation, differences between countries, the necessity of having stroke networks, and then the problems of designing trials to establish what the most effective drug is, whom it helps, and in what respect it helps. I would also like to thank the audience for their thoughtful questions and comments. Finally I would also like to thank the sponsor of this Symposium, Janssen-Cilag for their support. We may conclude that acute stroke therapy research has grown from early infancy to late infancy but not yet into early adulthood. I would propose that we have this discussion during each Annual European Stroke Conference in the coming years.

The promising results of intensified research

ACE and the Vascular Wall – from Genotype to Therapy

Editors:

Detlev Ganten
Klaus Lindpaintner
Bertram Pitt

Contents

Cardiology
Editor: Alpert, J.S. (Tucson, Ariz.)
ISSN 0008–6312
Supplement issue: Vol. 86, Suppl. 1 (1995)
Included in subscription

ACE and the Vascular Wall – from Genotype to Therapy
Roche Satellite Symposium, 12th World Congress of Cardiology, Berlin, September 1994
Editors: Ganten, D. (Berlin); Lindpaintner, K. (Boston, Mass.); Pitt, B. (Ann Arbor, Mich.)
IV + 46 p., 16 fig., 9 tab., soft cover, 1995
SFr. 25.– / DM 30.– / US$ 21.75
Prices subject to change
DM price for Germany, US$ price for USA only
ISBN 3–8055–6154–7

Fields of Interest: Cardiovascular System; Nephrology; Pharmacology

KI 95204

KARGER